Apocolyptic Pharmacy

Apocolyptic Pharmacy

A PRESCRIPTION TO AVOID DISASTER

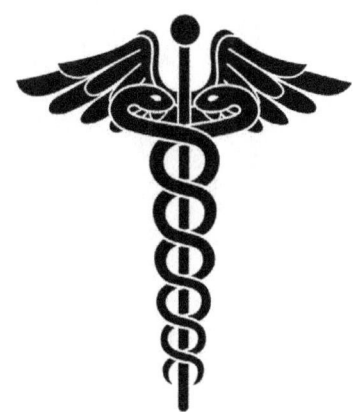

Steven C. Ohliger, Registered Pharmacist

ISBN: 1511465050
ISBN 13: 9781511465052
Library of Congress Control Number: 2015906056
CreateSpace Independent Publishing Platform
North Charleston, South Carolina

I wish to personally thank the following individuals, who without their contributions and support, this book would have not come to light in its present form. To my wife, who not only supported me in my efforts and helped format the interior, but also single-handedly designed the cover. To my parents, Steven & Judy, for meticulously editing the manuscript and supporting my endeavors.

Contents

Introduction

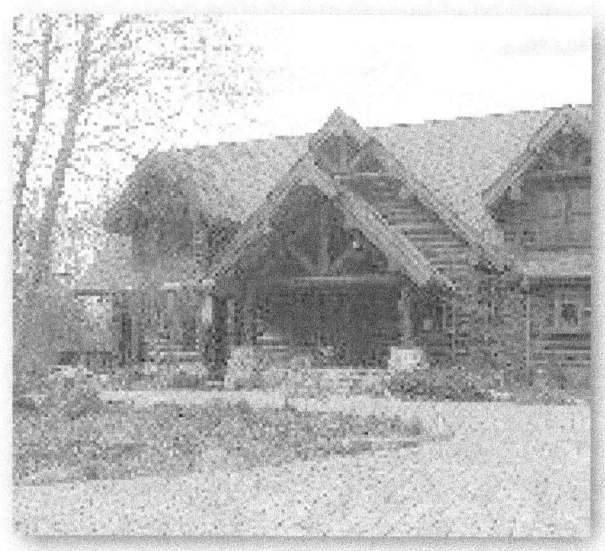

FOR THE PAST TEN YEARS, Tim Rupert had been working hard to prepare for what he believed to be an inevitable disaster. "Hoping for the best but preparing for the worst" was his motto. With so much going on in the world—the threat of a foreign invasion on US soil, an EMP, a terrorist biological or chemical attack, a collapse in the US economy—Tim had made sure he and his family were ready for anything.

Engaged in a successful career, he leveraged his 401(k) account and purchased a remote cabin far away from any major metropolitan areas. Fortunately he had the opportunity to work from home, which allowed him to continue earning money while at the same time spending time investing in upgrades to his property.

To begin with he had secured a two-year supply of dehydrated food. Then, over the next few years, he slowly built his provisions by adding renewable sources of food, such as rabbits, goats, chickens, and a large heirloom garden. Learning to harvest seeds from his garden, Tim had the knowledge to continue and expand his food harvest each year. Tim and his wife became proficient in preserving their food by becoming skilled in both canning and dehydrating techniques. They were equipped to produce more than enough food for their family for as long as they needed to.

In addition to obtaining fresh, unadulterated water from a natural spring on his secluded property, Tim installed a solar-powered pump to access his deep well in case the grid went down and his spring dried up. Several ponds on the property ensured they would always have an abundant source of water for his family, his animals, and his garden. Additionally, in the past couple of years, he built a rain-catchment system that stored runoff rainwater from his roof in several below-ground five-hundred-gallon containers.

The cabin was also equipped with at least two sources of electricity. Mounting multiple solar panels on his roof with an automatic sun-tracking system, he stored electricity in forklift-sized batteries. Backup power from several wind generators ensured that his family would never be without the conveniences of modern-day living. He had enough power to run any appliance in his home and could probably supply his neighbors' electrical demands as well. For heat Tim had a large wood-burning furnace that would easily keep his home warm during the cold winter months.

Finally, Tim gradually collected enough ammunition to match his growing collection of firearms. Training to be proficient in the use of all of his weapons, he and his family also took tactical training classes. They were all ready for any would-be invaders trespassing on their property.

Tim thought he was well prepared and was confident that he and his family would survive and thrive in a post-apocalyptic environment. So when the end finally did come, he was neither shocked nor fearful of the days ahead. He knew they were as ready as anyone could possibly be.

Two weeks after the fall of society, and after the initial rioting and violence had emptied out the local stores, his family was living with all of the comforts of their previous lives. Nothing could go wrong. Then, exactly twenty-one days after the collapse of society, Tim was carrying firewood across his property, and he collapsed.

Since the medical system had disappeared along with the government, there was no longer a hospital, doctor, or pharmacy available. Tim's prescription blood-pressure medication had run out the previous week. With nothing to keep his skyrocketing blood pressure under control, Tim's heart was working overtime until it finally exceeded its capabilities, and he suffered a mortal ischemic heart attack. Lying on the grass, Tim's last thoughts were how he had failed his family by not preparing adequately for the smallest and most overlooked essential area for maintaining life. He would not enjoy the fruits of his numerous plans and hard work because he had failed to take care of his own health.

Like Tim, many people either neglect or forget the importance of being able to continue a prescription regimen after a collapse of modern-day society.

Preparing for an upcoming major disaster may seem daunting and overwhelming. You have to think about food, shelter, water, security, heat, energy, and the list goes on and on and on. Starting small and gradually adding to your preparation plan, you continually accumulate more supplies and provisions. But it seems that no matter how many measures you take, there are always so many additional tasks that need to be done. With such a long to-do list, it may be easy to overlook something that seems small and insignificant at the time but is vitally important, and without it all of your best-made plans could crumble...just like Tim's. The chain in preparedness is only as strong as its weakest link. Fail in one critical area and the lifeline will ultimately break.

To underscore people's lack of knowledge concerning the importance of prescription medication preparedness, the next time you run into someone who shares your point of view (another prepper), ask him or her the following questions:

1) How much food, in months or years, have you stored?
2) How much water, in months or years, do you have access to?
3) What steps have you taken to protect you and your family (self-defense)?
4) Do you have plans for bugging out (or in)?
5) How much of your prescription medications, in days or weeks, do you have in the event that the medical system collapses?

I expect that most people have a good handle on where they stand on questions one through four. These are the most-pressing concerns for the majority of preppers, and they have already been working on plans for those essential items. Most all prepping books cover these areas ad nauseam. But I can almost guarantee that very few people have given any thought to the fifth question. They might look at you with blank expressions on their faces. The answer, or the lack of an answer, to question number five shows the inadequacy that *we all have* in a prescription-preparation strategy. Therefore my hope is to provide adequate information to start to fill in the gaps—to increase people's knowledge in the area of medication. My goal is to equip people so they can form action plans to protect their health in the event of a crisis. Finally, this book should help provide sufficient tools so we can better manage our own prescription-medication preparations.

CHAPTER 1

Why Am I Writing This Book?

LAST YEAR I HAD THE opportunity to attend a local conference on preparedness, which included many interesting and informative lectures. It seemed that the various classes covered almost all areas of preparedness. The learning opportunities were endless. There were an exhaustive amount of training classes, and my only disappointment at the end of the seminar was that I could not possibly attend all of them. For future conferences I have a growing list of lectures I would definitely like to attend.

At the conclusion of the seminar, while I was waiting for my wife to finish a late-running course, I happened to run into a mutual friend of ours. This friend and her husband have really taken the preparedness movement to heart. With expertise in the areas of dehydrating and canning, they have a vast supply of food stored up. They've also planted a large garden and an orchard for renewable food. As far as having an adequate supply of water, they're very fortunate to have a nice spring on their property. They have various other preparations that make me envious. In some ways both she and her husband seem far ahead of my own preparedness plans. So, with that in mind, I was surprised to find a grievous deficiency in their plans.

As she and I talked, she expressed her growing concern to me. Knowing my occupation she confided in me that she was worried about her supply of prescription medication. After a major collapse of society, she knows her medication would be difficult if not impossible to procure. The lack of this particular medication would have adverse effects on her overall health. It could be life threatening. She also told me that she felt there was a lack of information available regarding this specific area of preparedness (prescription medication). This reminded me of when I had read a very well-known fictional (but plausible) story in which an EMP knocks out the electrical grid and devastates the nation. In this book the main character tries to obtain insulin in order to continue to treat his daughter's diabetes. He initially is able to get a few vials from a failing pharmacy, but then they eventually run out, and his beloved daughter dies due to the inability to treat her medical problem.

Turning back to my friend, I empathized with her fear and anxiety, and we parted ways. Initially I didn't have the opportunity to give it much attention. What could I do? But like a smoldering ember, her problem continued to burn away in the back of my mind. Like a nagging mosquito, the issue kept buzzing around in my head until I finally tried looking around at the various resources available. I searched for any information on the availability of prescription medication if there came a time that pharmacies were unable to stay open. I scoured the Internet for any available information; I looked for books, manuals, and pamphlets. Surprisingly there was little information. I was shocked.

In the rare situation I did find anything pertaining to prescription medication, professionals knowledgeable in the area was lacking. I am in no way discrediting the various authors' works; some have done extensive research and written well-put-together articles. But the information available was not very informative, and it was scattered throughout different articles. Sometimes there was a little paragraph by one person here and then another document written by another writer there. No one has managed to collate all this important information together into one cohesive work. If you are anything like me, you like all of your ducks in a row. You want all of your fire-starting information in one place, all of your emergency medical treatment put together in another, and all of your food preservation together in one easy-to-find reference book.

Often the vast amount of information available merely touches on most areas of preparedness needs, though some do more extensively than others.

Without a doubt, when it comes to addressing prescription medications (if it appears at all), the information presented is just a blurb on a long list of items to stockpile. It is just a few words—"get prescription medications"—inserted between "get toothpaste" and "get toilet paper."

More attention is given to hoarding toilet paper (as possible post-apocalyptic currency) than is given to obtaining prescription medication. Toilet paper can keep you nice and clean, but having the proper medication can save your life. In addition to being buried in on a long list of "to get" items, no details 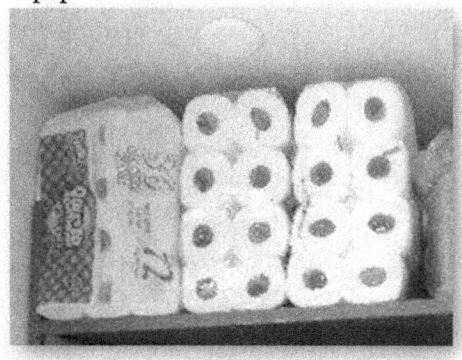 are given on *how* to obtain or preserve medication. Stockpiling medication, especially prescription medication, is extremely difficult under the watchful eye of the FDA. More so than toilet paper.

It seems that very few medical professionals are preppers. If there are medical professionals involved in the prepper movement, they are surprisingly silent about the lack of information available to the public on the subject of prescription medication. As it is now, there are very few resources and articles addressing the prescription-medication concerns after an end-of-the-world event. Regrettably this area has been long neglected. I want to change that.

What makes prescription-medication preparedness so increasingly difficult is the extreme regulation and oversight. Unlike food supplies and other survival gear, we cannot simply go out and purchase a two-year supply of prescription medication. Conversely, in the span of five minutes and a few clicks of the mouse, people can go online and order a five-year supply or more of dehydrated food. We can store up as much water as we have containers to hold it. We even have the freedom to purchase as much alcohol from the local liquor store as our credit cards allow. Some stores may have limits on the amount of ammunition we can purchase at one time, but we can still methodically acquire all we would ever need for hunting or self-defense.

In contrast, when it comes to obtaining something as important and vitally life sustaining as prescription medication, multiple roadblocks obstruct our paths. The federal government strictly regulates and controls the prescription-medication market under the watchful eyes of the FDA (Food and Drug Administration), state regulatory statutes, professional medical boards, the DEA (Drug Enforcement Agency), and the all-too-powerful insurance companies. It may seem easier to purchase the components for an explosive device than to acquire just one extra week of prescription medication.

Now, don't misunderstand me. I don't know of one pharmacist who doesn't want his or her customers to get their medication. But between the overly strict regulations and insurance companies that do whatever they can to avoid paying for your drugs, typical pharmacists finds that their hands are tied behind their backs. Nothing is more ridiculous to me than when I am not able to provide the customer with the medication the doctor originally prescribed. Fighting the insurance companies takes much of my valuable time. This is precious time that a pharmacist does not have because corporate greed wants the pharmacist to fill as many prescriptions as possible, with minimal help.

In practice I'm seeing more and more drugs that insurance companies are not willing to cover. Whatever bogus reason the insurance company has for not paying for a drug comes down to one and only one thing: money. Not only is the current trend extremely frustrating to pharmacists, but I'm sure physicians are tired of having to change their prescriptions because insurance companies do not want to cover expensive drugs. The truth is that not one pharmacist went to school to work in conditions like this. Every pharmacist entered the field to assist people with their medical care. But the grim reality is that corporations have cut the staffing so thin that most pharmacists have to work on their feet from dawn to dusk without even one break. The working conditions are akin to sweatshop labor. But I digress. Suffice it to say that pharmacists are on your side, but they have been castrated by the system.

Ultimately my goal here is to inform and educate you. I want to give you tips and strategies to maximize best your ability to survive if a major collapse of society occurs. There are things the government regulatory agencies and insurance companies don't want you to know. They don't want you informed. They want complete control of your life, health, and prescription medications. But there are, at least for now, loopholes you may be able to utilize to your advantage. In order to take the upper hand, and if you are to use these strategies to your benefit, you need to be organized and be able to plan ahead. If you are involved in the preparedness movement, these skills are already part of your everyday life. Just the fact that you are preparing, that you are reading this material, shows that you are already ahead of most people. However, the more people who know about these strategies and loopholes, the more likely it is the powers that be may catch on and try to close these holes.

Limitations

Controlled Drugs

I will not discuss strategies to maximize access to medications that are listed as controlled substances. Due to ethical standards, I cannot in good conscience expand on this topic any more than I already have. The risk of abuse or potential drug trafficking is too great. I do not wish to put my professional license at risk. I do not look good in an orange jumpsuit, so I'd like to avoid jail if at all possible. Besides, with the very strict oversight of the DEA, obtaining these types of medications is extremely difficult, if not impossible and illegal.

As a matter of fact, I use much of the technology available to me on a daily basis from the DEA and my state regulatory agencies to make decisions on whether or not I will fill prescriptions for controlled substances for certain patients. I have the ability to look up any and all controlled substances filled for a particular patient regardless of what pharmacy he or she got the prescription filled at. That's right. All controlled prescriptions are recorded electronically on a database that any pharmacist or physician can access. Think your prescription record is private? Think again. Unfortunately a few bad apples have spoiled it for the people who legitimately need controlled prescriptions.

This brings me to the next area of concern...

Privacy

As I've written above, the government tracks controlled medications extensively in an effort to keep the booming drug-trafficking problem under the guise of being held in check. You may be surprised to discover that more people than you think have access to your list of prescription medications.

Insurance companies maintain a list of your medications. Any time you have a prescription billed to your health insurance, it is recorded electronically and available to a vast array of people. You think your information would be restricted to professionals in the medical field. However, when you turn your rights over to the insurance industry, a wide variety of companies that claim they are using your information for legitimate research purposes can access your private health information. The sad part is that *they* determine who has the right to access your medical information. We have no input in who they can or cannot release our private information to because we waive that right when we join a plan.

Just by signing up with a medical-insurance company, you are authorizing them to release your information to third parties. Read the fine print of your insurance plan. Unfortunately we don't have much choice. It is a necessary evil. With the skyrocketing health-care costs today, we cannot afford to go without insurance coverage. We have to accept the companies' terms of use. They do not negotiate. Either we accept their terms, or we go without health insurance.

I can foresee in the future that the insurance companies will use our own private medical information against us. There will be a day when they base our policy prices on what is in our medical files. I can also see the day when they will deny us medical coverage and life-sustaining procedures based on our perceived risks. Welcome to the dreaded "death panels."

RECIPES

Second, the complicated system of manufacturing sophisticated medicinal medications will be a near impossibility in a post-apocalyptic environment. Disappointingly, to both you and me the process of making medicinal drugs is virtually out of reach. Some

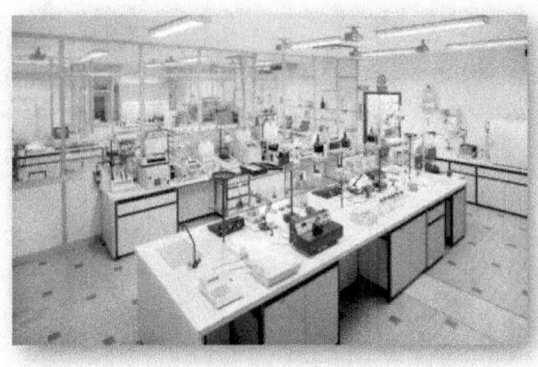

requirements are (but not limited to) complex laboratories, expensive laboratory equipment (centrifuges and sterile hoods), and extremely dangerous chemicals (such as hydrochloric acid, sulfuric acid, nitric acid, sodium hydroxide, and other potentially toxic or cancer-causing chemicals). Also an organic chemist or biochemist is necessary. If you are one of the rare people who has access to all of these elements, plus a standalone power grid, then you have the potential to be the richest person in a post-apocalyptic world. Or you may be able to barter your services for ample amounts of toilet paper.

You can manufacture certain chemicals, such as methamphetamine, in your basement. But again, this involves procuring ample toxic chemicals. Unfortunately the recipes, or chemical processes, for making prescription drugs are locked away in highly guarded drug-company safes. Additionally the end product must be analyzed and tested for potency, safety, and effectiveness before being used. Without complex laboratory equipment, this cannot be done.

Due to the highly improbable, virtually impossible ability to produce these medications even with a recipe, this is beyond the scope of this book.

ALTERNATIVE MEDICATION

I will address alternative or replacement medication later. But for now I cannot and will not endorse any herbal supplement or medicinal plant for use in treating a problem. Unless I have studies, or at least multiple personal testimonies, of the safety and effectiveness of a supplement or natural treatment, I will not mislead you into believing a method is viable when it may not be. Endorsing a product would require massive research, data analysis, and putting my stamp of approval on it. It is a huge undertaking to study all of the different claims and collate the information into a book. However, it may be a great proposal for a sequel.

DISCLAIMER

(To make the lawyers happy…)

The tips and strategies that I am about to describe are HYPOTHETICAL ONLY and for entertainment purposes only. They are only for extreme situations such as if a catastrophic event occurs and access to medical care, pharmacies, and hospitals is impossible. This book is not designed to and does not provide medical advice, professional diagnosis, treatment, or services to you or to any other individual. Medical information changes constantly. Therefore the information in this book should not be considered current, complete, or exhaustive, nor should you rely on such information to recommend a course of treatment for you or any other individual.

Before undertaking a new health-care regimen, never disregard any professional advice. Reliance on any information provided in this book or reference material is solely at your own risk. The information, including but not limited to text, graphics, images, and other material contained in this book, is for informational purposes only. The purpose of this book is to promote broad consumer understanding and knowledge. It is not intended to be a substitute for professional medical advice, diagnosis, or treatment. Always seek the advice of your physician or other qualified health-care provider with any questions you may have regarding a medical condition or medical advice. Do not delay in seeking advice because of something you have read in this book.

Now that that is over with…

My Credentials

You may already be asking yourself, "Who is this person writing this book? What gives him the expertise and authority to write about prescription medications?" I would expect nothing less than for you to ask those types of questions, so let me tell you a little about myself.

I am a registered pharmacist in several states. I graduated from an accredited college of pharmacy with distinction and was on the honors list. I was also a member of Kappa Psi (a professional pharmacy association) and Rho Chi (an honorary pharmacy association). Employed in the field of pharmacy for more than twenty years, I have worked in different and varying roles in the profession, which include: retail pharmacy (chain drugstores), hospital clinical pharmacy, and mail-order pharmacy. In the course of my employment, I have accumulated significant knowledge of the inner working of this field and have seen how insurance companies and regulatory agencies operate. I by no means claim to have *all* knowledge on a certain subject, and I am continually reminded (especially by my wife) of how much I still have to learn.

CHAPTER 2

Common Myths

MYTH #1

"After the collapse of society, I can still get my supplies at my local pharmacy."

The Truth:

Thinking that your local pharmacy will be up and running and fully stocked is like believing that your local grocery stores will be conducting business as usual after a collapse of society. This is not only naive thinking but also dangerous to your survival. After the panicking masses loot the grocery stores and clear out the merchandise, they will be heading to the pharmacy stores. Most pharmacies are a one-stop shopping area. In addition to stocking medical supplies, most pharmacies now carry a small portion of groceries, food, alcohol, and hardware. That and the fact that those stores contain prescription-strength narcotics is enticing to potentially desperate and dangerous people. It's like leaving young children in a toy store and telling them not to touch anything.

I'm sure that the lure of prescription (especially narcotic) drugs will be an irresistible draw for some. The only thing between them and the prescription department is a small gate that one can easily open with a simple crowbar. Once inside the pharmacy and high on drugs, they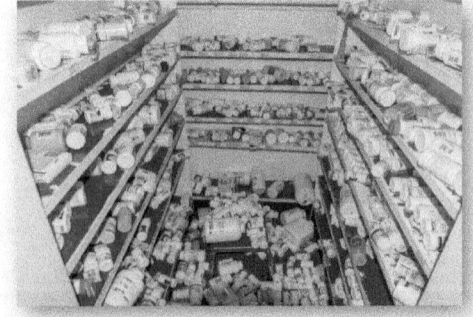

may be violent. People are unpredictable, as you may have witnessed during news clips of riots on TV. In crisis situations mobs of people go out and destroy and loot property for no reason. Rioters smash windows, start fires, and steal everything and anything they can get their hands on. Don't be surprised if the pharmacy is ruined after it is looted. The looters may have wanted only to take the narcotic drugs, but in the process they also took or destroyed your much-needed medication.

Pharmacy inventory can run in excess of a couple hundred thousand dollars. Upper management sees the drug inventory in pharmacies as negative profit and puts systems in place that try to minimize this while filling their pockets full of money. It pushes pharmacies to stock fewer and fewer drugs. The pharmacist gets in trouble, and corrective action is taken if he or she doesn't keep the inventory below a certain amount. The dollar amount that management allows keeps on shrinking year after year while the cost of medication goes up and up. This is the reason the pharmacy may not have your drug this month when they did have it last month. Like most retail stores, pharmacies are now on POS (point of sale) systems. The pharmacist is allowed to have only a certain quantity of medication on hand. Then, when that medication is sold through the register, the system is supposed to order more. Forced to keep such a low inventory of product is why, even now, they run out of medication quickly. A crash in the transportation sector will have a similar effect on the drugs as it will on the food on the grocery-store shelves.

In conclusion, pharmacies, even if they are open after a catastrophic event, will be prime looting locations. Not only that, but there will be a certain type of drug-seeking, addicted people that will make the environment even more dangerous. The prescription department will become a prime target. In all probably nothing useful would be left after the first wave of looters. Don't count on obtaining your medically necessary medication or medical supplies from your local pharmacy after the fall of society. There is no guarantee that your medication will be there. Acquire your medication now, before such a catastrophic event occurs.

MYTH #2

"After a major collapse of society, I won't need to take my medications any longer because I'll be eating healthier."

The Truth:

There is *some* validity to this particular myth since the typical American garbage-food diet will not be available after a collapse. Most fast-food chain restaurants will not be in operation. We have all heard of the country's wide obesity problem. The American diet is notorious

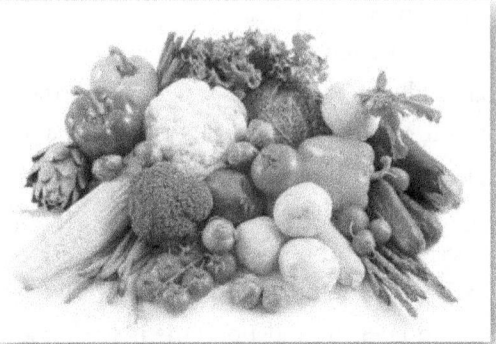

for being very unhealthy. The latest studies show that an average of 20 to 35 percent of the national population is obese. Unfortunately many medical complications arise from this high number of people who are overweight. More than *$190 billion* is spent on health care because of this epidemic.

Ironically there *is* an upside to a major societal meltdown. Our diets would most probably benefit as we are forced to eat more proteins and greens. And without the invasion of television or other electronic distractions like the Internet, social media, and texting, we will be required to develop more active lifestyles. A lot of physical tasks that technology, engines, and other laborers did will have to be done by the remaining survivors. Instead of putting the trash on the curb for someone else to pick up, we'll have to physically dig a hole and bury it. Instead of throwing something in the microwave, we'll have to sweat and chop firewood in order to cook. However, the benefits associated with increased physical activity and eating healthy does not entirely compensate for proper medication treatment.

First, not all medical conditions are due to poor diet and exercise. Proper diet and exercise are a good place to start and may help with diseases like type II diabetes, high cholesterol, high blood pressure, and many other conditions.

But they cannot cure every medical problem. For these types of diseases, proper medication administration is required to maintain health. Type I diabetes always needs insulin. Thyroid deficiencies will still need hormone replacement. And some heart and blood pressure problems are *not* entirely a result of poor eating or a lack of activity but rather due to other intrinsic hereditary causes. Just because someone is thin and eats well doesn't mean he or she does not have medical problems. Young marathon runners have dropped dead from heart attacks. People who eat only vegetables still die from cancer. Weight and exercise are not necessarily linked 100 percent with health.

Second, even if proper diet and exercise can reverse a condition, any change in health is not going to happen suddenly or overnight. As some of us may know, losing weight is not a rapid, easy process. It usually takes weeks or months before we notice any appreciable difference when we stand on the dreaded scale. Even if all of the fatty foods dropped off the face of the planet tomorrow, and we were left with only green, leafy vegetables, the process of losing weight still would take time.

Take, for instance, Tim in our fictional story at the beginning of this book. Tim may have been well on his way to losing weight and eating healthy. His physical activity had definitely improved since the collapse. However, he did not have enough heart medication to give him enough time to see if his change in lifestyle would help. Maybe if he had stockpiled enough, he could have given himself enough time to lose the weight. Then, in a couple of months, he could have tried to wean himself off of the medication to see if he could survive without it.

Third, it is almost never advisable to stop abruptly a prescription medication that your body has been depending on. In some instances suddenly stopping a medication can have devastating effects. In the story of Tim, he ran out of his prescription heart medication and was forced to suddenly do without. In his condition his body could not adjust to the sudden change. It would be like driving your car down the freeway at fifty-five miles per hour and coming to a complete stop (crashing) without slowing down. This would have detrimental effects on your body. So would completely and suddenly discontinuing a necessary medication.

You should research drug-specific recommendations for stopping your medication. Sometimes medications are eventually stopped by gradually cutting down the dosage over time and closely monitoring how the body reacts to less and less medicine. If all goes well and the body adjusts favorably to the lack of medication, then the drug can be discontinued. I never recommend anyone suddenly stop medication without first consulting with his or her physician. Prednisone is an excellent example of a medication that cannot be stopped suddenly without incurring disastrous effects.

In conclusion, while a societal breakdown will force us to eat healthier food and increase our activity level, we cannot rely upon this in and of itself for people to safely discontinue their own prescription medications. The underlying medical problem may not respond to a change in lifestyle. And it is never advisable to stop prescription medication suddenly without researching and/or discussing it with a medical professional.

Myth #3

"After I run out of my medication, I can forage substitutes from medicinal plants and herbs."

The Truth:

Foraging for plants can be extremely dangerous unless the forager is an expert in plant identification and knows which plants are toxic. According to the American Associate of Poisoning Control Centers, 50,579 people were poisoned by plants in 2010. And 5,912 people were poisoned just by eating the wrong type of mushroom. There were an estimated sixty fatalities from mistakenly eating poisonous mushrooms. Most people who came into contact with the poisonous plants sought immediate medical attention. But what will happen when there is no access to hospitals or emergency rooms?

Certain plants *may* have some medical properties (note emphasis), but there may be a lack of reliable sources or scientific studies to validate such claims. The FDA does not regulate statements on herbs and nutritional supplements, leaving room open to allow insidious people to make false claims in order to sell their products. Does anyone have the ability to read the two-second disclaimer that advertisers put on their TV ads promoting their special products? Who could possibly read the tiny print that flashes on the bottom of the screen for mere seconds while the miraculous benefits of the herbal supplement are being touted? Here is what the disclaimer says:

"These statements have not been evaluated by the Food and Drug Administration.
This product is not intended to diagnose, treat, cure or prevent any disease."

Regardless of your feelings about the FDA, the statement above can be translated in many cases as "our product does not work." I've been working in this field long enough to see overly hyped fad products come and then disappear as people spend good money before realizing it doesn't fulfill the promises that are advertised. Most of the "miracle" products are worthless. However, if you fall into the slim majority that feels that your supplement does work, count yourself as one of the lucky ones.

Read the ingredients, and make a rational decision before buying into the hype. All you're going to do is make someone else rich. For example, most "male enhancement" herbal supplements are simply vitamin B with some caffeine mixed in. Wow. (Note sarcasm.) One multivitamin and a cup of coffee may be less expensive.

I could easily tell you that African violets have anti-inflammatory properties without having anything to back up my statements. But try to prove me wrong. See? In the alternative medication industry, and believe me it is a multibillion-dollar industry, the burden of proof should be on the manufacturers to prove that their products work. They don't prove anything. The burden of proof should not be on the consumer to prove whether or not the products work. It is a "buyer beware" market. In addition to my false claim about the anti-inflammatory properties of African violets, if I did that with one hundred or more plants, I could publish a book and make lots of money because people would think I am an expert on medicinal plants even though I just made it all up in my head. Unfortunately live doctors do lie.

Like the saying "just because it's on the Internet doesn't make it true," you can add to the list "just because it is on a television ad or someone wrote a book about it doesn't make it true." That is not to say that all of the claims put out there are false, unfounded assertions. Just be careful. If it sounds too good to be true, it usually is. Research and check *everything.* Make sure the sources are credible and the claims are based upon solid facts. I have been around long enough to see most claims of so-called "miracle cures" swirl around before finally disappearing down the mysterious hole at the bottom of the toilet.

Certain plants may have *some* medical properties (note emphasis), but they also contain other toxic chemicals known as alkaloids. These alkaloids can cause bad side effects ranging from nausea, stomach upset, and vomiting to life-threatening effects like seizures and death. Without a lab to separate the good chemicals from the bad, you will be taking a risk ingesting the unhealthy parts of the plant.

Take, for instance, digoxin, which is most commonly used for congestive heart failure. Digoxin is derived from the digitalis plant. A common name for the digitalis plant is foxglove, which you may recognize for its historical use in assassination poisonings of the ruling nobility. Let's pretend the end of the world came, and your family member ran out of his digoxin

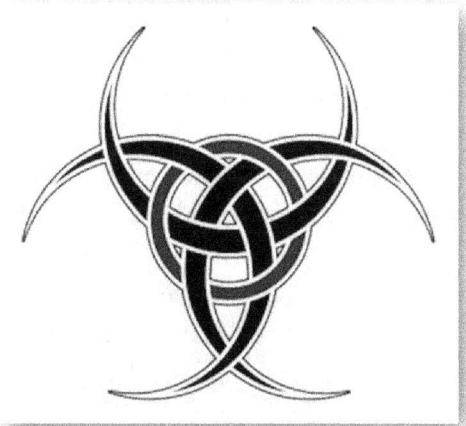

tablets. Let's also say that in anticipation of the collapse, you had the fortitude to plant a few foxglove plants. OK, now that your family member ran out of his much-needed tablets, you run out to the garden and stand over your plant. How much do you give? One leaf? Half a leaf? Just a nibble of the leaf?

Digoxin is a narrow therapeutic index drug (which we will discuss in more detail later). That means that if you give a tiny bit less than you should, it won't work effectively. But on the other hand, if you give just a little too much, your family member will have toxic side effects that could lead to death. With that in mind, ask yourself: How much of this plant would you give your loved one?

All medicinal prescription drugs are manufactured under strict quality controls in sealed laboratories. These labs are heavily regulated and must meet the government's good manufacturing practices (federal law with strict policies that labs must follow). The active medication is extracted from other potentially harmful chemicals and concentrated into a tablet or a capsule. When you ingest this medication, the pharmaceutical company is putting its liability on the line that the dosage is correct and that there are no other harmful chemicals in it. There is not this type of guarantee when you attempt to harvest the drug from your own plants.

When we hear the word *natural*, we immediately think it is good. Our brains have been wired that way due to the constant advertising campaign of the industry. Just because something is natural does not make it safe. Poison ivy is natural. Cyanide is natural, but the only condition it can cure is life. Alkaloids and digitalis are naturally occurring substances, and we've already discussed the possible hazards of these chemicals.

In conclusion, I am *not* saying that medicinal substitutes cannot be foraged from plants in an emergency. In fact if I had no other option, I would attempt to do so myself. However, the risks involved would lead me, at all costs, to try to obtain reliable prescription drugs before foraging became necessary. The guessing game in the proper amount of medicinal plants to give and the fact that there are also dangerous, toxic alkaloids in the plant would cause me serious concern. I would probably attempt foraging for replacement medicinal drugs only as a last resort.

CHAPTER 3

Acquiring Prescription Medication

As you may have guessed by now, obtaining prescription medication is the first and most difficult obstacle in trying to add to your supply stock. Learning to preserve your medication will be of little value if you have nothing to conserve. The strategies ahead will require both patience and meticulous planning. It is a slow process, but if the end of days comes, it will be well worth it. Again, the strategies are hypothetical, and all dosage/drug changes should be discussed with your physician.

Over a period of around five years when I was living in South Florida, I accumulated and stored my own personal medication using a couple of the methods listed below. At the end of five years, my wife and I decided to pack up our belongings and move to another state. Leaving my employer, I lost my health insurance, which covered my medication. When I moved from South Florida, I left my established physician who wrote prescriptions for my medication. Even so, I had enough of my prescription medication stored away that I had more than two years of medication stockpiled!

Once in my new state, I didn't have to rush to get a new physician. This was good since there was a three- to six-month waiting period for new-patient appointments. Despite that fact I was not frantically trying to get my medication at a new pharmacy with a new prescription drug plan. I cannot even begin to describe the peace and lack of anxiety I had concerning my prescriptions. Enough was stored away that I didn't have to worry about it.

Now I have a new physician, and I am working on rebuilding my stockpile in case of a future emergency or disruption in supply. Who knows what the future holds? Maybe I'll have to move again and reestablish my medical coverage. Or maybe an end-of-the-world event will occur, and the supply will be cut off. Either way my mind is completely at ease because I am confident that I am doing all I can to maximize my stockpile.

Now, you may be thinking, *Of course he has a good stockpile of medication. He's a pharmacist! He has unlimited access to prescription drugs!* That would be true, but I'm not that type of person. I hold myself to the strictest of standards and try to maintain a high integrity. I have never helped myself to anything that doesn't belong to me, and I do not fill any medications unless I have a legitimate and active prescription on file. Keeping myself above reproach, I don't even fill my own prescriptions. I have another pharmacist do it. I don't touch my drugs until I've purchased them from the pharmacy. Everything I have done in this book is above board, legit, and legal. You can do it too. I have never used my position to my advantage.

I know too many people who don't have even a week's worth of medication on hand in case of an emergency. Like living paycheck to paycheck, they live from refill to refill. They wait until the last possible minute to reorder their medication. If they are out of refills, and their physician doesn't authorize a refill quickly, or if the pharmacy has to order the medication, they have to do without. Talk about anxiety! There have been numerous times when I've seen panicking people who suddenly ran out of medication on a weekend or holiday. There is no excuse for that amount of poor planning. If they fail to prepare adequately for only one day without medication, what are they going to do when there is no longer access to pharmacies or hospitals?

When we were living in South Florida, hurricanes were a recurring threat every year during the summer months. The public would be told over and over again to have at least three days of food and water in case a hurricane hit and knocked out local resources. When a hurricane approached, we had at least five days to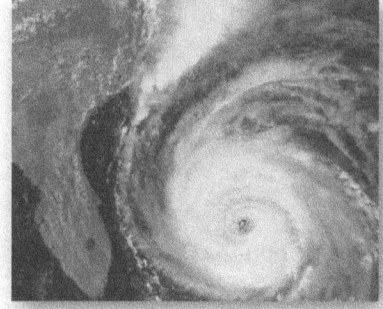

prepare. In the aftermath of the hurricane, it amazed me how many people were on the streets looking for food and water. It was simply incredible. The old saying is true: You can lead a horse to water, but you can't make it drink.

Before I dive into the possible strategies, I feel compelled to give a word of
warning. Do not use the words *stockpiling* or *hoarding* when dealing with
physicians, pharmacies, or insurance
companies. Even though these words do
not carry any negative connotations to
us, they will set off red flags with others.
People outside of the prepping community already think that storing up years
of food for the future is crazy. Trying to

accumulate prescription medications will set off multiple alarms with the medical community and the government. They'll most likely label you as a drug addict even though the medications we are talking about are not addictive, only life sustaining. Regardless, they will watch you like a hawk and possibly limit the amount of prescription medication you can store for the future.

I will list some of the strategies for obtaining prescription medication in my personal order of preference. I will start with the simplest and best and gradually work down to the more complicated. None of what I am going to discuss is illegal or unethical, although some regulatory bodies may frown on the practice. If you have reservations about collecting extra prescription medications and somehow think it is unethical, let me propose the following scenario.

The government has crashed, the economy has come to a grinding halt, and the remaining bad people are rioting, killing, and raping. Your fam-
ily is starving and will soon die without food. Your precious little child is weak with hunger and can barely move. Would you take food (steal) from the local grocery store? Would you break into an unoccupied home to raid the cupboards (robbery)? Or, if you managed to obtain some food for your

family, could you harm, even kill someone who is trying to take that food from you, knowing that if he or she succeeded your family would surely die of hunger? What lengths would you go to in trying to preserve your life and your family's lives?

STRATEGY #1: EARLY REFILLS

Have your prescription refilled the maximum amount of days before your next refill is due. Get it refilled as early as you are allowed. Sounds simple, right? There is one hurdle to getting early refills. If all prescriptions were dirt cheap and we bought them with cash, this would not be an issue. The major problem is that we rely on insurance to cover part of the cost of the medication. Without insurance, the cost of prescription medication is discouraging, if not impossible, for us to afford. If we require assistance to pay for our medications, then we have to play by the rules put forth by the insurance companies. And all of the companies put a limit to how early we can get medication refilled.

Fortunately the insurance companies do allow for us to get our medications early—a grace period. So there is a positive side of the giant medical industry…one. The companies realize we cannot always pick up our medication on the exact day that it runs out. For example, if we have thirty days' worth of medication, they know that due to life circumstances we cannot go to the pharmacy and pick up another supply exactly every thirty days. Due to weather, work, school, children, doctor appointments, and other scheduling issues, setting aside a specific day to visit the pharmacy every month is not feasible. The pharmacy may also need a couple of days to order the medication. Or the doctor may not have had a chance to authorize a renewal on the medication. Delays are unavoidable and should be expected. Surprisingly the insurance companies understand that we are all human, and they allow us to get a tiny bit more medication. That is because the risks involved if you to go without medications will ultimately cost them more in the long run if you experience problems. It all boils down to risk assessment.

Most health insurances, if not all, allow for early refills. A general rule of thumb (and this may differ depending on your particular plan) is that they will allow up to seven days early on a thirty-day prescription and twenty-one days early on a ninety-day prescription. To get the particulars on your own

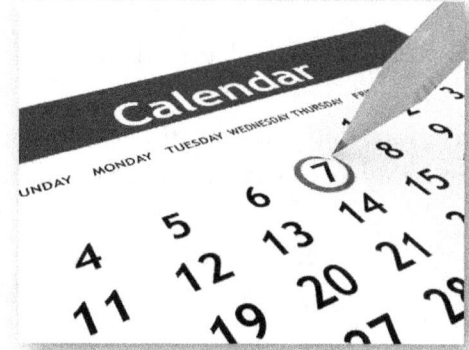

drug plan, it would be best to call their customer service department and ask them. The number is listed on the back of your insurance card.

Use this grace period allowed by the insurance company to your advantage. Refill all of your prescriptions as early as you are allowed. Let's examine two scenarios. In the first I will refill my medication only on the day that it is due to be refilled. In the second scenario, I will refill my prescription as early as I am allowed. For simplicity let's also pretend that every month has thirty days. In this first case, I am not a forward-thinking kind of person and just get my thirty-day supply of medication refilled on the first of every month. I also wait until the very last due day to pay my bills (and that is why I have a lot of extra late charges). Here we go. I have a thirty-day supply of medication, and I refill my prescription every month on the first when I am down to my last pill. Every month I get thirty days' worth of medication. Therefore, over a period of three hundred sixty days (about a year), I will have received three hundred sixty days of medication.

$$30 \text{ days} \times 12 \text{ months} = 360$$

Makes sense, right? Of course this also means that if some unexpected problem occurs, like the pharmacy had to order the medication, or I didn't realize that my doctor didn't give me any refills, then I'd be in trouble because I would not have any extra pills.

Now, if I had that same thirty-day supply, and I asked the pharmacy to refill my prescription seven days early each and every month, I would have received seven extra days of medication each month.

$$30 \text{ days} + 7 \text{ extra days} = 37 \text{ days of medication per month}$$

For each thirty-day month, I'd have thirty-seven days' worth of medication, or eighty-four extra days of medication over three hundred sixty days!

$$37 \text{ days' worth of medication per month} \times 12 \text{ months} = 84 \text{ extra days of}$$
$$\text{medicine}$$

This is almost three months' worth of extra medication that I can stockpile every year! In the first scenario I don't have any extra doses of medication and am at risk of going without my drugs if a problem occurs. In the second scenario, I have plenty of extra put aside for an emergency situation.

This strategy is currently the best-known way that I know of to accumulate a decent supply of extra medication. I have used this before, and it is the reason why I could afford not to worry about obtaining medication for more than two years. I am still using this strategy for a possible future emergency. It's all about being prepared.

At the present time, most prescription drug plans allow early refills. Like I stated before, if they let you, why not take full advantage of it? I need to add that only very rarely have I seen insurance companies try to limit early refills if they catch on to the fact that you constantly ask for them. I think I have seen this only once or twice over my career, and it was with a government plan. But if they get wise, they may start clamping down on early refills in the future.

There are some important things you must do to set this up and make it run smoothly. First, as I've mentioned before, find out exactly how many days early your insurance company will pay for your medication.

Second, before you sign up with your local pharmacy for an automatic refill plan (i.e., a plan in which your prescriptions are refilled automatically each month), find out how their computers are set up to fill. Unfortunately, at some stores they refill your prescription automatically every thirty days (for a thirty-day prescription), which defeats the purpose of trying to get your medication early.

I've had most success with mail-order companies. I know that a lot of people do not like mail order for one reason or the other. However, I was very happy with the service. I set up my account to refill my prescriptions automatically and automatically contact my doctor if I ran out of refills. Then, like clockwork, I received my medications in the mail. They routinely refilled my prescriptions as early as the insurance plan would allow, and I received them shipped for free in my mailbox. I didn't have to remember to refill my medication manually or spend the time and gasoline to pick it up from my local pharmacy.

Third, and this is vitally important, be sure your physician writes out your prescription to meet your needs. People usually miss this important step because the prescription writing comes at the end of the office visit and happens as your doctor is finishing and walking out the door. There are two things you need the doctor to do for you:

1. Before your physician starts the prescribing process, ask him or her to please write for a thirty-day (or ninety-day) supply based on what your drug plan pays for. (It is easier to ask for a ninety-day supply because even if your drug plan pays for only a thirty-day supply, the pharmacy can always reduce the quantity dispensed. However, the opposite is not true. Your pharmacy cannot legally change your prescription from a thirty-day supply to a ninety-day supply without contacting your physician for approval.) Physicians are sensitive to their patients' finances and will most always write for the maximum that the insurance will pay for.

2. If your physician is willing to write for a year's supply of your medication, ask for PRN refills. *PRN* stands for "as needed." This means that instead of being limited to a specific amount of times you can refill your prescription, you are allowed to refill your prescription as needed for twelve months. All prescriptions expire and are not refillable after twelve months from the date they are written (except controlled substances, which expired after six months). Believe it or not, there is a big difference between PRN and eleven refills. If your doctor writes your prescription for the original fill (the medication you receive when you first turn in your prescription) plus eleven refills, you would receive twelve months', or three hundred sixty days', worth of medication. Then you would need a new prescription.

30 days X 12 fills (the original plus 11 refills) = 360 days' worth

However, if on the same prescription your doctor writes for the original filling plus PRN refills, you can receive fifteen months' worth of medication per year. That is because when you refill your prescription early each month, you'll actually be using fourteen refills per calendar year until that prescription expires.

I know this can be confusing to understand. Let's say you take full advantage of refilling your prescription as early as you are allowed every month (i.e., seven days early). If the doctor wrote your prescription on January 1 for eleven refills, and it is good for one year after it is written, you could get it filled on January 1, January 23 (first refill), February 16 (second refill), March 9 (third refill)...until September 13 (twelfth refill). Your prescription has not lasted a full year.

If the same prescription had PRN refills, you could continue getting it filled past September 13 and up until December 31, when the prescription actually expired.

Finally, and most importantly, get yourself set up so you can order your refills each month as soon as your drug plan will pay for it. Get a wall calendar and mark the days, set up your computer to alert you, or utilize an automatic refill plan; just make sure that you take full advantage of this strategy. Use it now before the insurance companies start to close the loophole.

Saving up three months of medication per year might seem pathetic and slow compared to how much food you can put up in a year. However, with all of the regulation and oversight in the prescription drug market, this is probably the best and least difficult way. If you plan accordingly and are disciplined in getting your medication filled early, you can accumulate a decent amount over a few years. It is better than the alternative of having nothing saved.

Strategy #2: Dosage Change

In my initial template for this chapter, I was going to place all dose changes, including dosage increases and dosage decreases, under this heading. However, due to the specifications of each topic, I am compelled to split it up into three different sections in order to explain each one adequately. The following strategies require that you put on your thinking cap and sharpen your basic math skills.

Let's say you go in for a scheduled office visit with your physician. For whatever reason, your doctor decides either to increase or to decrease the dosage of your medication. He or she writes you a new prescription for the new dosage. Now, what do you do with all of the medication you still have? What about that prescription for the old strength that's still on file at your local pharmacy? Although I cannot recommend what you should do, I can tell you what I might do in the same situation.

INCREASE IN STRENGTH

Your physician may decide that the current strength of your medication is not sufficient, and you need to be on a stronger dosage. This happens quite often and is usually because your physician starts you on a small dose, sees if it works for you, and increases the dosage as needed. He or she wants you to start out taking the smallest dose available to treat your condition because with larger doses comes a greater chance of side effects. If he or she does increase your dose, what can you do with the smaller dose of medication?

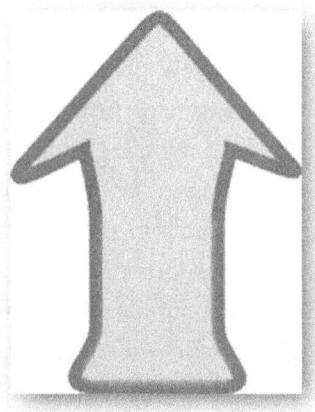

Let's pretend that my doctor changes my medication from twenty-five milligrams a day to fifty milligrams a day. I get the new medication—the fifty milligrams—filled immediately. I can use up my twenty-five milligram dosage while building up extra of the fifty milligram dosage. I use up my old twenty-five milligram dosage by taking two (two twenty-five milligrams equal one fifty milligrams). It's the same dosage my doctor wants me to be on. My old prescription will last only half as long because I'm taking twice the amount per dose, but I am stocking up on the new strength by not taking it. Once I've used up the older dosage of medication, I can switch over to the new dosage.

As a precaution, and in order to avoid mistakes, I would take a felt-tip pen, cross out the old directions, and write the new directions on my old bottle of twenty-five milligram pills. Instead of the directions reading "take one tablet daily," I would handwrite, "Take two tablets (fifty milligrams) daily." I would include both the number of tablets and the total dosage in milligrams (or whatever units the medication comes in). This way there is no question in my mind of what my dosage currently is.

If the doctor increases my dosage to seventy-five milligrams, I would write, "Take three tablets (seventy-five milligrams) daily." For one hundred milligrams, I would write, "Take four tablets (one hundred milligrams) daily," and so on.

Let's go back to my original prescription above, for the twenty-five milligrams dose. I've told you what I would do with my old prescription that I have at home. What about the old prescription for twenty-five milligrams that's still on file at the pharmacy? Unless the physician writes somewhere on the new prescription for my fifty-milligram medication that this is a new dosage or instructs the pharmacist to discontinue the twenty-five milligrams, my old prescription will still remain active on file at the pharmacy. It will continue to remain active and refillable as long as it hasn't expired (one year from the date it was written) or the refills haven't run out.

Therefore it is possible for me to get not only my new fifty milligram prescription but also the old prescription for twenty-five milligrams refilled. Most pharmacists will take a patient at his or her word if he or she tells the pharmacist he or she is on both strengths. The only special precaution I would take as a patient is that each time I got the old prescription refilled, I would make absolutely sure to update the directions on the bottle immediately after bringing it home. That way there should be no confusion about my current dosage. Then I would continue filling both strengths for as long as I could. I should be able to accumulate extra medication for emergencies using this strategy.

But what if my medication is a fifty-milligram tablet, and my physician increases the dosage to seventy-five milligrams? That means that I will have to take one and a half of the fifty-milligram tablets in order to get the seventy-five milligram dose. Obviously you cannot cut a capsule in half, so this method pertains only to tablets. Although the math isn't all that difficult, I need you to refer to the information on cutting tablets in the following section before even thinking about attempting this.

Decrease in Strength

Although it's not common, your physician may decide to decrease the dosage of your medication. This may occur because you are experiencing side effects of the drug, and a lower dose may help, or possibly the drug is working very well, and the physician has determined that you can try to take less. The strategy below will work only for tablets. Capsules cannot be cut in half.

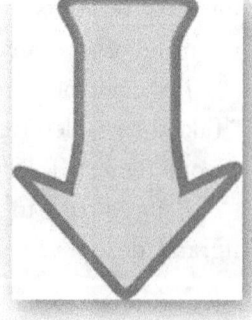

I recently had my doctor decrease a dosage of my medication from fifty milligrams to twenty-five milligrams. I had almost one hundred eighty days of the fifty-milligram tablets that would have otherwise gone to waste. There was no way I was going to throw them away. I went out and purchased a pill cutter and cut all of the fifty-milligram tablets in half. Similar to what I did with the previous dosage change, I took a felt-tip pen, crossed out the directions on my old bottle, and wrote, "Take one half tablet (twenty-five milligrams) daily." It took me a little time, and my cuts weren't too precise, but now I have three hundred sixty doses (one year's worth) of my medication. This is in addition to the new prescription of twenty-five milligrams that I am currently getting filled. As an added bonus, I can still get my old prescription for fifty milligrams refilled from the pharmacy until it runs out. It just means that I'll have to cut more tablets.

Precautions for Cutting Tablets

#1: Narrow Therapeutic Index Drugs

We need to discuss drugs with a narrow therapeutic index. In terms that are easy to understand, this means that the drug dosage is so sensitive, there is little room for dosage changes. Too little of the drug and it doesn't have its medicinal effect on the body. Conversely, a little too much of the drug and there may be toxic effects.

Each drug has a therapeutic index, which is the range, from the smallest to the largest, in which a dosage is effective. The difference is that some drugs have large therapeutic indexes. That means that dosages are not that critical. Drugs with narrow therapeutic indexes mean that the dosage is critical to maintain the level in the body between a minimum effective dosage and a minimum toxic concentration. Some examples of drugs with narrow therapeutic indexes (according to the FDA) are digoxin, theophylline, lithium, phenytoin, and warfarin. A complete list of these medications is available on www.FDA.gov. These drugs are exempt from our discussion, as the dosages are specific and need to be taken exactly as prescribed.

A better analogy would be this. Imagine riding a bicycle down a paved, two-lane highway. The left side represents the lowest dosage possible that still has the intended effect. The right side of the highway represents toxicity. Unless you are drunk or completely incompetent, it is fairly easy to ride your bicycle and stay on the road. This represents most drugs to a varying degree. Some roads might be slightly wider, some narrower. The distance from one side to the other is the hypothetical therapeutic index of the medication.

For a drug with a narrow therapeutic index, imagine riding the same bicycle down the same road, but you have to keep your tires between the double yellow lines running down the center of the road. A slight drift to the left and the medication has no effect. A wobble to the right and you risk toxic drug side effects. Normally your physician will be testing your blood levels periodically if he or she puts you on a drug with a narrow therapeutic index to ensure that your dosage is correct. I highly advise not using any of these strategies on medications that have sensitive dosages.

#2: Cutting Tablets

Cutting tablets, even with a pill cutter, is not an exact science. It is almost impossible to cut a tablet in half, even if it is a scored tablet, so that one side has precisely the same amount of medication as the other half.

Certain tablets *cannot* and *should not* be cut, especially medications that are sustained-release, delayed-release, enteric coated, controlled-release, etc. These tablets are specifically designed to release the medication over a certain period. If you cut 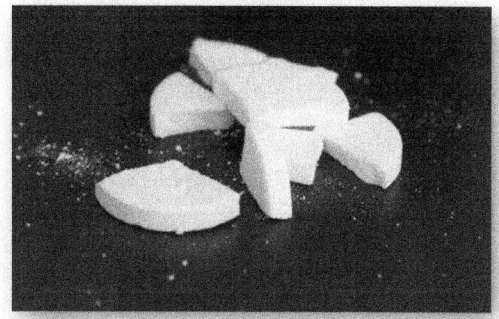 these tablets, a "dose-dumping" syndrome will likely occur. When the tablet's integrity is altered, it can release the full dosage of the medication all at once instead of gradually over time. This will result in unsafe high levels of medication in the body. It can be toxic. Avoid cutting these types of tablets at all costs. For a full, updated list of medications that should not be cut, refer to www.ISMP.org (Institute for Safe Medication Practices). They publish an excellent reference of all medications that should not be cut or crushed.

Obviously, neither capsules nor gelcaps can be cut either with any accuracy.

STRATEGY #3: MEDICATION CHANGE (WITHIN THE SAME CLASS)

If my physician decides to change my medication to another medication within the same class, I have a few options, however limited. I am specifically referring to two different medications that are in the same therapeutic class, such as two calcium-channel blockers, two beta-blockers, two nonsteroidal anti-inflammatory agents (NSAIDs), etc. In this situation the two medicines are very similar. Examples of two different medications that are in the same therapeutic class are naproxen (Aleve) and ibuprofen (Motrin). They are two different drugs, but are both NSAIDs. They both have very similar chemical structures, indications, actions, and side effects.

For this you have to know what classification your old and new prescriptions belong to. The patient-information paperwork that you receive with your prescription usually states the classification. If there is any question, simply ask your pharmacist or physician if your old medication and new medication are in the same therapeutic class.

Now, the strategy. First, I would ask my physician if he wants me to switch to the new medication right away or if I could use up my remaining stock of old medication and then switch to the new one. If it is OK for me to use up my old medication first, I would still get my new medication filled right away and use strategy one—early refills.

If my physician wants me to switch right away, I would store my old medication (see the preserving medication section later) for safekeeping. I may not ever have to use the old medication, but at least I would have something if there comes a time when there is no access to a pharmacy. If I run out of my new medication, I may consider taking the old medication. In my mind it could be better than taking nothing.

As an additional benefit to saving my old medication, I could use it as a bartering tool. Who knows? Maybe someone else will need the medication I am no longer taking.

STRATEGY #4: MEDICATION CHANGE (OUTSIDE OF SAME CLASS)

If my physician changes my medication to a completely different therapeutic class, my options are even more limited. An example of this would be a change from a beta-blocker to a calcium-channel blocker. These medications are completely different in chemical structure and actions.

If this were the case, I would store my old prescription for future bartering. Only in extremely desperate scenarios would I consider taking the old medication. If an end-of-the-world-as-we-know-it event occurred, I ran out of my stockpile of current medication, and there were no viable alternatives available, I may try to take the old medication. It would be a personal choice, and then I would have to weigh my decision based on the risks of not taking it.

Strategy #5: Obtaining Medication Out of the Country

Although the United States does not allow importation of prescription drugs from outside of its borders, more recently the government has taken a stance of "don't ask, don't tell." According to the FDA website: "Although importing unapproved prescription drugs is illegal, the FDA's guidance on importing prescription drugs for personal use recognizes that there may be circumstances in which the FDA can exercise 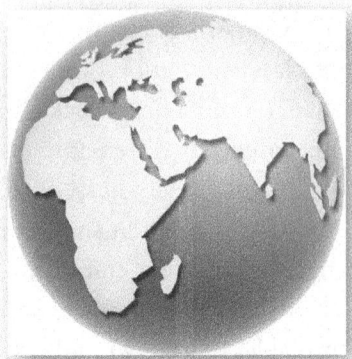 discretion to not take action against the illegal importation." Further, it states:

> The current policy is not a law or a regulation, but serves as guidance for FDA personnel. The importation of certain unapproved prescription medications for personal use may be allowed in some circumstances if all of these factors apply:
>
> - if the intended use is for a serious condition for which effective treatment may not be available domestically
> - if the product is not considered to represent an unreasonable risk
> - if the individual seeking to import the drug affirms in writing that it is for the patient's own use and provides the name and address of the U.S.-licensed doctor responsible for his or her treatment with the drug or provides evidence that the drug is for continuation of a treatment begun in a foreign country
> - if the product is for personal use and is a three-month supply or less and not for resale, since larger amounts would lend themselves to commercialization
> - if there is no known commercialization or promotion to U.S. residents by those involved in distribution of the product.

There are strict limits to what you can order. First, no controlled substances may cross the border. This is illegal and would be considered trafficking.

Second, purchasing medications outside of the United States can be only for the individual obtaining the medication. Third, the quantity purchased can be only a maximum of a ninety-day supply of medication.

Another huge risk of ordering from outside the United States is the quality of medication that you will receive. Are you actually getting what you think you are? Again, it is a "buyer beware" market. The prescription-drug industry is a multibillion-dollar business and everyone, good and bad, wants a piece of the pie. There have been multiple cases of people receiving counterfeit drugs. The counterfeiters are so good, they have duplicated the size, color, and shape of the original medication, so it is almost indistinguishable from the real product. As technology continues to improve, these false products are becoming so like the brand-name products that only a chemical analysis can differentiate a real drug from a false one. Even if a counterfeit operation is discovered in another country, there is little that can be done about it since the company is outside of US jurisdiction.

There have been instances where Tamiflu® ordered from India has arrived with only talc and acetaminophen in the capsule, neither of which is an active component of Tamiflu®. Drugs imported from other countries have been tested and have totally different ingredients than what they are supposed to have. Some medications have even been laced with haloperidol, a powerful antipsychotic medication. People who took this medication required emergency, life-saving medical treatment. In other instances the medication ordered had the right ingredient, but the strength was incorrect.

If you decide to order medication from outside of the United States, do your due diligence. Order from a well-known, reputable company that is an established institution. I would not order from companies based in countries like India, China, or any third world country. If I had to obtain medication outside of the United States for personal use, I would first search Canada or Western European countries like France or Italy.

There are some obvious red flags that show up when ordering from an unsafe company:

- They send you medications with unknown quality
- They send medication from an unknown manufacturer.

- They do not provide a way to contact them by phone.
- There is no address for the company or the distributor.
- They offer prices that are incredibly cheaper.
- The product you receive looks different, tastes different, or smells different from the original medication you take.

Multiple Prescriptions/Physicians/Pharmacies

I have not listed this as a strategy because regulatory agencies consider this practice fraudulent, illegal, or at the very least unethical. They are in the process of cracking down on polypharmacy (using multiple pharmacies) and doctor shopping (obtaining multiple prescriptions from multiple physicians).

Some of these practices would include things such as faxing in your prescription to a pharmacy or multiple pharmacies and then getting the original prescription filled at a different pharmacy. Normal pharmacies do not permit a patient to fax in their own prescription, but in some cases Internet and foreign pharmacies will allow you to do so.

Another practice that people use is obtaining multiple prescriptions for the same medication from different physicians (doctor shopping). To keep the practice hidden from regulators and insurance companies, these people go to different pharmacies and pay cash for the medication. Since a prescription is classified as a legal document, using a prescription in this manner is considered fraudulent and may incur criminal charges.

CHAPTER 4

Animal Antibiotics

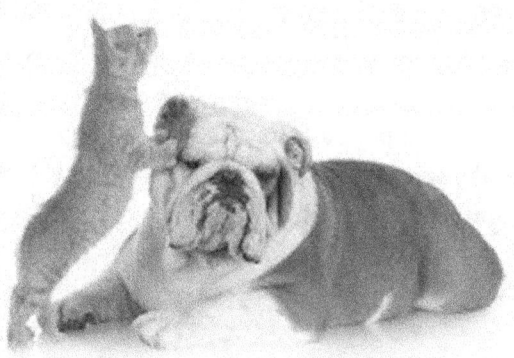

DUE TO THE EXTENSIVE INTEREST in obtaining animal antibiotics for human use after a collapse of society, I will devote this section to this specific topic. In a post collapse scenario, any infection can be life threatening. A cough, cold, or small cut can turn deadly. This is why proper planning should also include trying to acquire antibiotics now, while they are still available. Once an end-of-the-world event occurs, these medications will be impossible to find. The demand for antibiotics will skyrocket, making them more valuable than gold—but not quite as valuable as toilet paper.

Fortunately, or unfortunately, most physicians will not write a prescription for antibiotics unless they deem it necessary. It is fortunate because over-prescribing of antibiotics is resulting in the emergence of so called superbugs. I have been in the industry long enough to know that we are losing the war on these microscopic bugs. New strains emerge each year, and the pharmaceutical industry has not come out with any significant antibiotics in the past ten to fifteen years. Superbugs are bacteria that have mutated to be resistant to certain antibiotics that they used to be sensitive to. We can partially blame the mutations into these superbugs on physicians prescribing too many antibiotics. This has led to many responsible doctors in the community to prescribe antibiotics only when necessary. This extreme caution in prescribing antibiotics is necessary but unfortunate for those of us who would like to store some for emergency situations.

I can still find fish antibiotics available on the Internet, but I have noticed that my local pet stores are no longer carrying them. Growing up, I used to purchase fish antibiotics without a problem. (Yes, I did have a fish tank). It makes me wonder if government regulation has led to stricter control of the sales of these items. I have been in several pet stores recently and have not been able to find any antibiotics that humans can use. I have also walked up and down the aisles of farm-supply stores and not found anything that could be of use. They do have a few injectable products that have similar antibiotic ingredients, but as you will read later, injectables are not very stable and do not keep long. They also require special administration, which an inexperienced person cannot do.

Unable to procure any medicine from local stores, I am forced to turn to the Internet. From my research, the best way to acquire antibiotics for human use is to buy them over the Internet, and the best products for this are fish antibiotics. There are a few precautions one must diligently observe.

Buying medication over the Internet is risky. Everybody wants a piece of this multibillion-dollar industry, and they don't care about you. They just want to line their pockets with cold, hard cash. There are a lot of unscrupulous vendors out there who think nothing of falsifying products. Research the company. Don't just use the information available on their website, because they can advertise anything they want you to read. Search the company through other websites. Read consumer reviews. You may discover that the company has a US address, but the actual products are made and shipped out of Pakistan. Absolutely avoid any company outside of the United States.

You don't know what you are getting. Although not completely risk free, any company selling fraudulent products inside the country faces stiff monetary penalties, felony charges, and jail time. Make sure you are buying from an established, reputable company. Finally, when you receive the product, find a drug identifier (available online) and make sure that the color, size, and pill markings match the description of the drug.

As with all medications, people may have allergies to certain medications. If you take a medication and experience a rash, itching, or hives, you may have a mild to moderate allergy to the drug. Trouble breathing or heart palpitations indicate a severe allergic reaction that requires immediate medical treatment. An allergy can develop overnight or over a long period of time. It may happen when you take your first dose, or it may start after you've taken your fifteenth dose. Either way you should stop taking the medication and make a special note of which drug you had a reaction to. Avoid any other medication in the same classification category. For example, if you are allergic to penicillin, avoid any medication in the penicillin family, such as amoxicillin, ampicillin, dicloxacillin, and anything else that ends in "-cillin." You may even need to avoid cephalosporins because there is a 10 percent chance that if you are allergic to penicillin, you are also allergic to cephalosporins.

Mild or moderate allergic reactions can be treated with diphenhydramine (brand name: Benadryl®). The usual dosage on the package of twenty-five milligrams is one to two capsules or tablets every four to six hours. For an allergic reaction, I would take two. It will cause drowsiness, so no drinking alcohol, driving, or operating equipment. A severe allergic reaction may require injectable epinephrine administration.

If a collapse of society occurs and there is no longer access to physicians or hospitals, you may have to determine when you should or should not take an antibiotic. As a precaution I would avoid overusing antibiotics. I would not run to my stock every time I sneeze or feel bad. Using too much will lead to antibiotic resistance, like we discussed before. Overuse will also deplete your stockpile quickly, and you may find yourself without anything when you truly do need it. Underuse by not taking enough antibiotic or stopping it too soon will also risk the formation of superbugs. Generally, depending on the antibiotic medication, they should be taken for a minimum of seven to fourteen days. Additional resources are available for more extensive reading: *Where There Are No Doctors, The Nursing Drug Handbook, The PDR (Physicians Drug Reference)*, and *The Merck Manual* are all excellent references that can assist in determining if an antibiotic should be used and what kind in various circumstances.

Finally, not all veterinary drugs can be used safely in humans. Use only the products with the active ingredients on the list below. These are antibiotics that physicians are currently prescribing for human use.

As a pharmacist I am not allowed to diagnose or treat people. This is a realm specifically assigned to physicians. Therefore, I am going to list the antibiotic medications, the usual and customary doses in normal patients, and any special precautions. I am not prescribing the medications or instructing you on how to take them. I am just supplying the information. It is not an all-inclusive list but just the basics.

There are different dosages depending on the infection you're treating. This is just a baseline, a starting point, for use only when medical professionals are unavailable. Dosage adjustments may be needed in special conditions, including but not limited to liver or kidney disease, age, or any special conditions. These medications should not be taken if there has been any previous allergic reaction to any component within the classification of the medication.

In dosages expressed in milligrams per kilogram, you will need a calculator. To calculate the body weight in kilograms, take the weight (in pounds) and divide that by 2.2. For example, a one-hundred-eighty-pound person is eighty-one kilograms.

$$180lbs / 2.2 = 81 \text{ kg}$$

Then multiply the dose by the kilogram. For example, if the dosage is five milligrams per kilogram, you would first determine the body weight in kilograms (eighty-one kilograms in our example) and then multiply by the dosage per kilogram:

$$5 \text{ mg per kg} \times 81 \text{ kg} = 405 \text{ mg}$$

If the dosage is expressed in milligrams per kilograms per day, then a further calculation is required. The dosage you have calculated will be the total dose *per day*; you must further divide it by how many doses you are giving that day. Take the example above. If the dosage is five milligrams per kilograms per day given every eight hours, then we must divide the total daily dose by three (every eight hours = three times per day).

5 mg per kg per day every 8 hours =
405 mg per day (given every 8 hours) =
135 mg every 8 hours

Note: The availability of fish antibiotics seems to be disappearing. Many are being discontinued at this moment. I would recommend getting at least a few rounds of each antibiotic (enough to dose two to three times). Make sure that the expiration dates are at least a couple of years or more. Be prepared to pay more for these medications. They cost a lot more than their human counterparts, and health insurance, pharmacy plans, and other discounts do not apply.

Also remember that just as not all human medications can be used in animals (the chemicals are toxic to animals), not all animal antibiotics or other medications can be used safely or effectively in humans.

Amoxicillin or Ampicillin

Class:	Penicillin
Uses:	Many bacterial infections, including bronchitis, pneumonia, urinary tract infection, ear, nose, and throat infection gonorrhea, and tonsillitis.
Precautions:	Do not use if previous allergic reactions, liver or kidney disease, asthma
Normal Adult Dosage:	
	500 mg by mouth every 8 hours for 7-10 days
Normal Pediatric Dose:	
	4 weeks–3 months: 10-15 mg/kg (maximum 500 mg per dose) every 12 hours
	3 months-12 years: 10-25 mg/kg (maximum 500 mg per dose) every 12 hours
Availability:	Fish antibiotic: 250 or 500mg capsules

Cephalexin

Class:	Cephalosporin
Uses:	Bacterial infections including respiratory, skin, ear, and many others
Precautions:	Do not use if previous allergic reactions, liver or kidney disease, intestinal or stomach disorders, diabetes
Normal Adult Dosage:	
	250-500 mg by mouth every 6 hours for 10-14 days, or 500 mg by mouth every 12 hours for 10-14 days
Normal Pediatric Dosage:	
	12.5-25 mg/kg every 6 hours for 10-14 days, or 12.5-25 mg/kg every 12 hours for 10-14 days
Availability:	Fish antibiotic: 250mg or 500mg capsules

Ciprofloxin

Class:	Fluoroquinolone
Uses:	Most bacterial infections
Precautions:	Do not use if previous allergic reactions, liver or kidney disease, concurrent use of tizanidine or blood thinner, prolonged QT interval, any heart rhythm disorder, muscle or nerve disorder, tendon, arthritis, or joint problems, seizures, epilepsy, brain tumor or disorder, myasthenia gravis, Type II diabetes, or have low levels of potassium
Normal Adult Dosage:	500-750 mg by mouth every 12 hours for 7-14 days
Normal Pediatric Dosage:	(should not be the first choice due to adverse reactions in children) 1-18 years old: 10-20 mg/kg (maximum 750 mg per dose) every 12 hours
Availability:	Fish antibiotic: 250mg or 500mg capsules

Clindamycin

Class:	Lincosamide
Uses:	Multiple bacterial infections, malaria
Precautions:	Do not use if previous allergic reactions or allergy to yellow dye, liver or kidney disease, intestinal or stomach disorders, asthma, eczema, stop taking if persistent diarrhea
Normal Adult Dosage:	150-450 mg by mouth every 6 hours for 10-14 days
Normal Pediatric Dosage:	Weight 10 kg or less: 37.5 mg every 8 hours Weight more than 10 kg: 8-25 mg/kg per day, in 3-4 divided doses
Availability:	Fish antibiotic: 150mg capsules

Doxycycline

Class: Tetracycline

Uses: Acne, bacterial infections of the eye, intestinal tract, urinary tract, gum disease, Chlamydia, Gonorrhea, **Typhus, Cholera** and many other bacterial infections

Precautions: Do not use if previous allergic reactions to tetracyclines or sulfites, liver or kidney disease, asthma, concurrent use with seizure, isotretinoin, or blood thinner medication, do not use in children or pregnancy. May cause sun-sensitivity.

Normal Adult Dosage:

        50-100 mg by mouth every 12 hours for 7-10 days

Normal Pediatric Dosage:
(not recommended)

Availability: Fish antibiotic: 100 mg powder packets
        Bird antibiotic: 100 mg tablets

Erythromycin

Class:	Macrolide
Uses:	Bacterial infections including respiratory, skin, ear, and many others
Precautions:	Do not use if previous allergic reactions. Can interact with many drugs – need to research if your medications react. Caution in liver or kidney disease, prolonged QT interval, any heart rhythm disorder, myasthenia gravis, low levels of potassium or magnesium
Normal Adult Dosage:	250-500 mg by mouth every 6 hours
Normal Pediatric Dosage:	40-50 mg/kg/day divided every 6 hours (maximum of 2000 mg per day)
Availability:	Fish antibiotic: 300 mg powder packets

Metronidazole

Class:	Nitroimidazole
Uses:	Bacterial infections of the vagina, skin, stomach, joints, respiratory tract, and other infections
Precautions:	Do not use if previous allergic reactions, liver disease, stomach, intestinal, or blood cell disorder, nerve disorder, or epilepsy

Normal Adult Dosage:

7.5 mg/kg by mouth every 6 hours for 7-10 days

Normal Pediatric Dosage:

30-50 mg/kg/day every 8 hours for 10 days

Availability:	Fish antibiotic: 250mg or 500mg

Penicillin

Class:	Penicillin
Uses:	Many bacterial infections
Precautions:	Do not use if previous allergic reactions, liver or kidney disease, asthma, or bleeding disorder
Normal Adult Dosage:	
	250-500 mg by mouth every 6 hours for 14-21 days
Normal Pediatric Dosage:	
	125-500 mg by mouth every 6 hours for 14-21 days
Availability:	Fish antibiotic: 250mg or 500mg tablets

PRESERVING PRESCRIPTION MEDICATION

Like stockpiled food and water, prescription medication has a limited shelf life. The second law of thermodynamics states that everything in the universe decays over time. Simply look at our cars, our homes, and our own bodies. They all require attention and maintenance to slow the inevitable process of breaking down. It was a tedious process to obtain a supply of medications, so you would want to preserve it as long as you possibly can. There is debate and controversy over just how long drugs are good for, and we will touch on the pharmaceutical industry and expiration dates a little later. But for now there are steps we can take that will increase the chances that our medications will last longer.

First, let's all agree that almost everything, except certain snack cakes, has a limited shelf life. Canned food is good for only a certain amount of time. Even freeze-dried, expertly packed food can guarantee only ten to fifteen years of quality. Medications definitely have shelf lives too.

Expiration dates

Expiration dates on medications are required by law. There is a slight difference between the expiration dates on medications and the expiration dates on food products. The difference is that a medication expiration date is a date selected by the drug manufacturer beyond which they cannot guarantee the potency and/or safety of that medication.

For instance, a drug manufacturer makes a medication and ships it from the facility. Once made, the potency of the medication degrades over time depending on a number of factors. Like a new automobile driven off of the car lot starts losing value immediately, a medication starts to lose potency. For the sake of simplic-

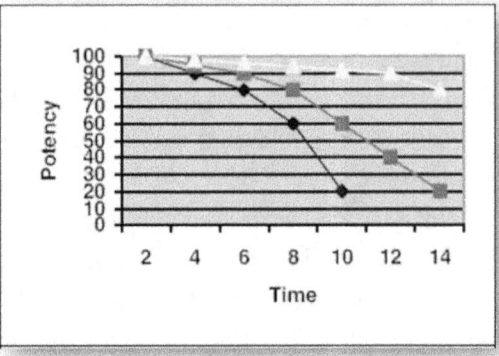

Expiration Chart

ity, let's assume that the manufacturer has just made MyDrug#1. At this point in time, we expect that the medication is 100 percent potent. After one year some of the components of the medication have degraded, and now it is 99 percent potent. The next year it is at 98 percent of its original potency. The next year it will be 97 percent and so on. Once the medication reaches less than 90 percent of its original potency, the FDA classifies it as expired, and it should not be used.

This is what the FDA says and what I must abide by as a medical professional. I cannot recommend or suggest that anyone take a medication past its 90 percent (expiration) date. Does this mean the medication will work at 90 percent and not at 89 percent? Will it still work at 80 percent? From my perspective the medication is still 80 percent good, but I still cannot tell anyone to continue taking it.

Hypothetically, if society came to a crashing halt and I had some medicine that I needed that was only 65 percent potent, I may still take it thinking that I am at least getting some benefit. I might even take two, thinking that I could get 100 percent of the benefit. But that, again, is an individual decision that must be made.

For further information on the acceptable potency of medications beyond their expiration dates, I would refer people to the SLEP (Shelf Life Extension Program), which was created by the FDA for the Department of Defense. In some circumstances the *active* component of the prescription medication was still 90 percent effective for twenty-eight to forty years after the expiration date. More information on the SLEP reports can be found online (US National Library of Medicine and the National Institutes of Health).

That being said, there are certain medications I would absolutely not take or recommend taking past the expiration dates. These include all liquids, sprays, seizure medications, nitroglycerin, injections, some sustained-release medications, and drugs that have narrow therapeutic indexes. Again, I would encourage someone who is considering expiration dates to research the safety and efficacy of his or her own particular medication. Know your drug inside and out!

Now I would like to address the controversial subject of pharmaceutical expiration dates. There are a growing number of people who subscribe to the theory that the pharmaceutical companies place early expiration dates on their products to increase sales. The conspiracy theory goes that if a product expires quickly, then it must be replaced (purchased by the consumer) more often than if the product had a longer expiration date. This, theoretically, would increase sales of the product and improve profits for the company. While this may be possible, I do not consider this very probable. (Irate complaints can be sent to me at Steve@IdontCare.com.)

The reason I don't subscribe to this particular conspiracy theory is that as an insider in the industry, it does not make much sense to me. The amount of product in every medicine cabinet does not compare to how much of the product is sitting on the shelves in all of the stores, pharmacies, and warehouses. We are talking about tons of product that has not been sold. When the product expires, it is sent back to the manufacturer for credit. The amount sent back for credit greatly outweighs the one bottle that may be sitting in a few medicine cabinets. Therefore the pharmaceutical manufacturer is losing money overall on expiration dates. The shorter the expiration date, the more product is sent back to the company for credit. Therefore shorter expiration dates mean less profit overall for the company.

Why is there a discrepancy between the expiration date placed on a medicine and the actual expiration of the product?

First, there are safety and liability concerns. When a medication is submitted to the FDA for approval, the drug manufacturer must include multiple studies of the potency degradation of that product. Let's take my previous example of MyDrug#1. The drug manufacturer may have ten studies (most probably they are required to have more) of the degradation of potency over time. Again, for simplicity, let's assume that the ten studies came back indicating that the drug reached 90 percent potency at two years, ten years, ten years, ten years, eleven years, fifteen years, fifteen years, sixteen years, twenty years, and twenty years respectively. Guess which expiration date the FDA would require to be used? Think it is the average? No. The answer is two years. Yes, even though some studies would support at least twenty years, the drug manufacturer would have to put a two-year expiration date on the product. Not only would the FDA require it, but the drug manufacturer would want to. Suppose that someone picked up a bottle of MyDrug#1 that had a five-year expiration date printed on it and took the medication. A good lawyer researching the degradation studies would find that one report says the drug is good for only two years. The manufacturer would be at fault and have to pay out exorbitant fees and settlements.

The drug manufacturers not only use early expiration dates to appease the FDA, but in most instances they also put in buffers for liability reasons. If a drug expires in five years, the manufacturer may put a three- or four-year expiration date on it just to ensure that the medication doesn't expire before they claim it will. Also, the drug manufacturer cannot guarantee how the customer handles the medication once he or she takes it out of the store. Sometimes we may do things that will seriously jeopardize the expiration dates on our own medications. More on that and techniques we can use to preserve our medications later.

Additionally, both the state regulatory agencies and large corporate retail pharmacy's procedures require pharmacies to put expiration dates on your prescription vials. The usual and customary expiration date is exactly one year after the prescription is dispensed. The stock bottle that your medication comes from may have a five-year expiration date, but once the drug is put in the vial and sold, the pharmacy is required to put at maximum a one-year expiration date on the prescription. The exception is if the medication actually expires in less than one year; then the pharmacy must put the exact expiration date on the vial. The one-year maximum expiration date is mostly for liability protection and the fact that we, as consumers, jeopardize the potencies of our own medications. We can be the worst enemies of our medications' expiration dates.

One additional thought before we move on. To date, I am not aware of any specific reports of dangerous human effects linked to taking expired medications. Only one incident occurred with tetracycline, which is no longer available on the market. In 1963 a report was filed maintaining that a patient had ingested expired tetracycline and it caused a renal tubular problem called Fanconi syndrome.

CHAPTER 5

Dosage Forms

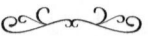

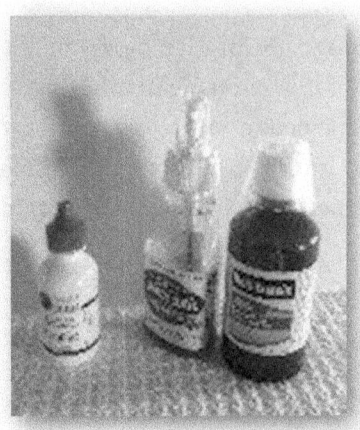

THE FORM IN WHICH A medicinal drug is available also affects its stability. Generally liquids and injectables are the least stable of all of the forms available and do not have long expiration dates. Some of these even require specialized storage or refrigeration to keep them viable.

Next most vulnerable are creams, ointments, and other topical products. Their expiration dates should be stamped or printed on either end of the boxes. If you no longer have the box that the product was sold in, the expiration date is stamped on the tube crimp (opposite the cap where the product comes out of the tube). You may need good light or even a magnifying glass to see the tiny date stamped into the aluminum.

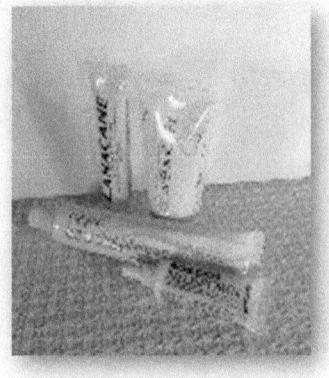

Moving toward more stable products, I would consider capsules (and gelcaps) to be next on the list. While highly stable on their own, capsules still do not have the integrity of hard tablets. The soft outer shell of a capsule is usually made out of gelatin and has the ability to 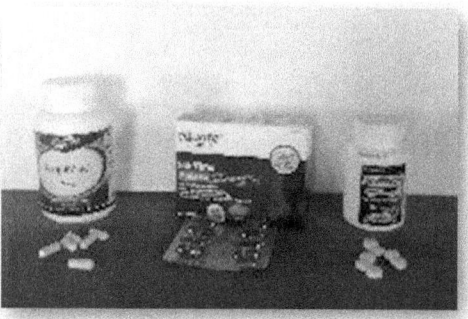 attract and absorb moisture. A capsule is specifically made this way so that when it reaches your stomach, the outer shell dissolves and releases its contents. Degradation can begin if the capsule is exposed to moisture in the air before being used.

Finally, the best dosage form available for stability is a tablet. The hard outer shell is best for resisting the effects of degradation. Tablets are not foolproof and still need protection from expiration-causing elements, but they are the best for our purposes.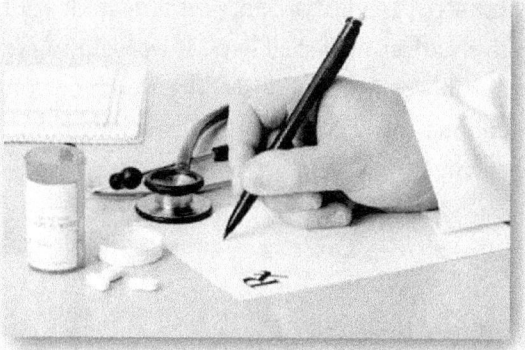

Overall, if a medication is available in some or all of these different forms, I would ask my physician to prescribe tablets when available.

CHAPTER 6

Enemies of Drug Preservation

LIKE FOOD AND WATER, MEDICINAL drugs have common enemies that negatively affect their shelf lives. If we want to preserve our medication as long as we possibly can, we need to address each one of these adversaries and learn how to counter them. We will use the acronym MALT to identify and categorize our enemy:

M—moisture
A—air
L—light
T—temperature

Any one of these enemies can seriously compromise the expiration date and integrity of a stockpiled medication. We must combat each one to preserve our medications to their maximum potentials.

Can you guess what the worst room in your house is to store your medications (excluding your garage and attic)? What room has all of these enemies? You are right—your bathroom! And the bathroom is where most people keep their medicines. The humid air from the bath or shower, plus the change in temperatures, makes the bathroom the worst room to store your medications.

Guess what the second-worst room in your house is? Probably where you also keep medicine stored—in your kitchen. Again, changes in temperature and humidity are the main culprits jeopardizing your medications' expiration dates.

MOISTURE

Moisture is a common enemy of anything we are trying to preserve. It is in the air we breathe. Without some form of water dissolved in the air, our lungs would dry out, our skin would crack, and we would require continuous hydration in order to live. But the moisture is bad for drugs. Too much wa-

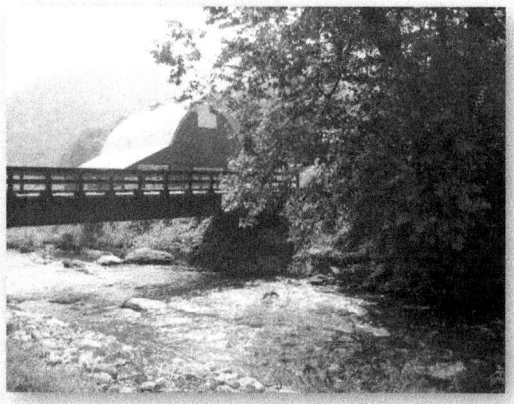

ter in the air reacts with the surface of the medication and causes it to degrade. It affects capsules more than tablets, but the hard tablets are still susceptible to the effects of moisture.

To combat the enemy moisture, it is best to store medications in an area that has low humidity. Although it's not really practical, the absolute best place would be inside of a cool, dry root cellar. However, any other room in your house would do as long as the humidity doesn't fluctuate like it does in a bathroom.

Another thing to consider is the container that the medication is in. If at all possible, use the manufacturer's bottle. The cap usually contains a good, airtight seal that prevents moisture from getting inside. Alternatively, look at

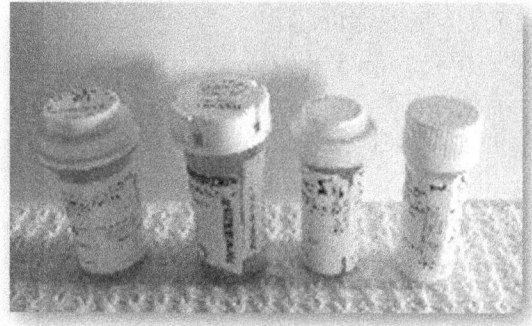

your prescription vial. Some may be better than others to keep moisture out. To test your pharmacy's vials, use an old, empty prescription vial and place the top on securely. Fill your sink with water, and submerge the vial. If you see bubbles escaping, your vial cannot block the invasion of moisture. Consider placing your vials in some sort of sealable plastic bag for temporary use.

For long-term storage (for medications you are not using any longer and want to put up for future bartering), take an additional step and seal them inside a Mylar bag. Again, the outside needs to be labeled with the full name of the medication, its strength, the date you packed it in the Mylar bag, and the expiration date. I would use one Mylar bag per prescription. Putting multiple medications in the same sealed bag will be confusing later on.

I'm sure I don't have to say this, but I will anyway. It is common sense. When you open your bottle or vial and take your dosage of medication out, limit any influx of moisture by immediately closing your bottle or vial. Always securely cap your bottles and prescription vials after use. Make sure the caps are on tight (but not too tight). If you have a large stock bottle of medication, like a thousand-count bottle of ibuprofen bought at your local deep-discount store, consider placing it in smaller bottles. Make sure the smaller bottles are labeled properly with the full drug name, expiration date, and lot number and the date you put the medication inside. By opening only the smaller bottle when you need your medicine, you are reducing the exposure of your large-bottled supply of medication to the elements. Ideally, have one smaller, labeled bottle in which you place fifty or one hundred tablets. Once it's empty, refill it from your larger stock bottle. That way, instead of exposing your main supply to the elements fifty to one hundred times (every time you want to take ibuprofen), you would be exposing your main supply only ten times over the life of your medication.

If you open your medication for temporary use, such as for putting a week's supply in a pillbox, try to minimize the time that your stock bottle remains open. Keeping medication for a short period (one to two weeks) in a pillbox is OK. Just make sure the container closes well and snaps. Replace the container when it worn and doesn't close securely. Avoid drastic or extreme changes in environment.

Also, remember to rotate your stock! Just like food, you need to keep the earliest expiration date up front so you use that up first. Organization is your best friend. Every time you buy more products from the store, check the expiration dates and place them appropriately in your storage area, with the earliest expiration dates in front and the latest dates in back. Also, when purchasing your medications, make sure to look through all of the bottles on the store shelves. Employees are trained to rotate the store's stock as well. Usually the best-dated products are in the back!

AIR

Air, or more specifically oxygen, is our next enemy that we are going to tackle. Oxygen oxidizes (of course) products. Oxidation is what turns your fresh-cut apples brown and rusts your metal. Molecularly, oxidation occurs when oxygen exchanges electrons with the product with which it comes into contact. I will save you grief by avoiding 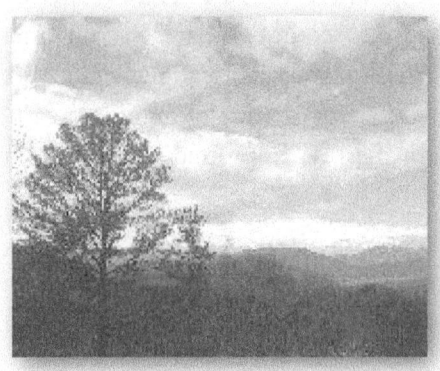 going into the exact chemical reaction that occurs. I've tortured you enough already with the previous math. Let us just assume that oxygen will eventually have a negative effect on your stored medication.

To combat the effects of air on your medications, use the same precautions as stated previously to prevent moisture from getting to your drugs. Keep your medication in the original bottle if possible, and open it only briefly to take out your medication. Make sure the seal is tight. Rotate your stock.

LIGHT

Light has a negative effect on many things, including your prescription medication. Notice how the sun bleaches out the paint on the roof of an old car or damages skin as a person ages. The same thing can happen to your medication. Ever wonder why you get your pre- 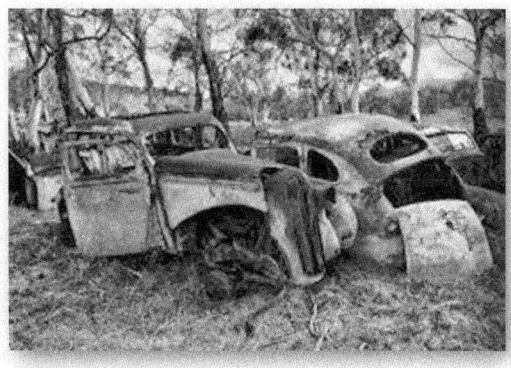 scription medication dispensed to you in an amber vial? The amber vial filters out harmful UV light.

To combat the effects of light, follow the same steps outlined above for both moisture and air. Go ahead and take an additional step of placing the medication in an amber vial. Remember, if you can see inside your vial, some light is going through the plastic (or else you wouldn't be able to see inside). Store your medication in a dark room or closet. If that's not possible, place your vials in a black plastic zip bag or opaque box. That will guarantee that no light is penetrating your medication. Then, for easy reference, place a sticker on the outside of the bag with the medication name, the date you put it in the bag, and the printed expiration date. Don't forget to rotate your stock.

Light also has the negative effect of fading out the actual prescription label. There is nothing worse than going into your stock and finding that you cannot read or identify an older prescription you had saved. Some pharmacy labels hold up better than others. The easiest and most inexpensive way to prevent your prescription vials from fading and becoming unreadable is simply to place a strip of clear plastic tape over the label. Make sure it is clear tape! The printed type will remain readable for many, many years. Do this with all of your prescription medications when you first bring them home, and you'll never have a problem.

Temperature

I saved the most-destructive enemy for last. Extremes in temperature can degrade your medication very quickly. In fact you may want to plan ahead if you know you are go-ing to purchase medications and have multiple errands to run. The inside temperature of

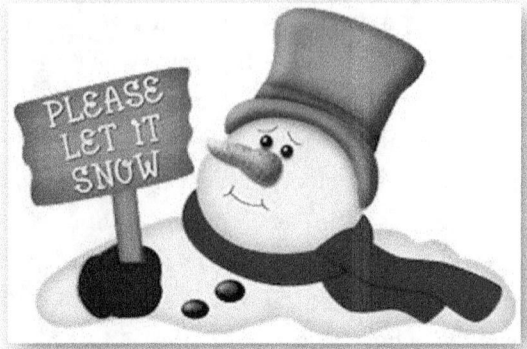

your car can reach in excess of one hundred degrees or more. Medication left in the car at that temperature will be damaged. Just as you wouldn't leave a child, a pet, or ice cream in that environment, don't leave your medication in there to suffer. In minutes heat can greatly reduce the expiration date of your medicine by *years*! Don't take a chance. Bring an empty cooler, and place your medication inside, or better yet make sure your medication purchase is your last stop on the way home.

Also avoid storing medications in rooms that have large temperature fluc-tuations, like the bathroom or kitchen. Although not necessarily practical, the absolute best place would be a dry, cool root cellar. Even though this area is not feasible for all of your drugs, you may consider storing your bulk bottles and other medication that you don't plan on using for a while there. If you have medications you are not using any longer and just want to keep on hand for emergencies or bartering purposes, a root cellar would be a perfect storage area.

If you successfully fight against these four enemies of expiration dates, you have the ability not only to preserve your vital medications, but possibly to extend their shelf lives beyond what the manufacturers have printed on the bottles.

CHAPTER 7

Over-the-Counter Necessities

COME WITH ME ON A short trip to the local pharmacy. Don't worry about your car keys; I'll drive. I even have a list of what you might consider purchasing. These are the OTC (over-the-counter) items you need to stock up on. They don't require prescriptions, and you can purchase as much as you need. Don't worry; it won't hurt your wallet too much. Well, maybe just a little. You are not going to clean out the store but buy just a few items from each category to make sure you are well stocked and prepared in case the store is not open for business in the future.

"How much are you going to buy?" you may ask apprehensively as you ride in the car. To this I answer that it's not a question of how many pills you are going to buy; it is a question of how much, in time, you are going to plan for. If money is not a limiting factor, you will purchase as much as you can for the maximum amount of time. If you can afford it, you will buy the amount needed up to the expiration date. If a nonprescription product has a five-year expiration date, you will purchase five years' worth of it. Then, as you use up your stock at home, you will replace it. As you replace what you used up, you will always have sufficient quantity. Remember, you need to continue to rotate your stock, putting the first-expiring product in the front. If you are diligent about rotating your supply, your medicine will never go out of date. You will have a five-year supply of the medicine at all times. I know that the initial cost might be hefty, but nothing is ever cheaper than it is today. Prices, along with inflation, keep increasing.

If you are constrained by a limited budget, I recommend getting a year's worth of medication. It may not seem like much, but a year's supply is a good start. In my estimation, a two-year supply of medication would be an ideal starting place. It seems like a good compromise. Now, you need to figure out how much a year's supply is. That I cannot answer. That is up to you. Try to think back and see how much you have used of a certain OTC product in the past year. How much headache medication have you taken? Are you taking your vitamins on a regular basis? How long does one tube of antibiotic cream last you? These are questions you have to answer for yourself.

OK. We are finally at the pharmacy. I put the car in park, and we go inside and grab a cart. If disinfectant wipes are offered, be sure to wipe down the bar where you put your hands to push the cart around. This metal-and-plastic bar happens to be the dirtiest thing you'll touch today. Shopping carts are notorious for harboring viruses and bacteria.

The following are the fundamentals. I firmly believe that the products listed below are the necessary building blocks for a well-rounded stock of OTC preparations. If you have any other special things you use, such as hemorrhoid, female, or ostomy products, go ahead and get them. If you get the following items, you are off to a good, solid start.

Aisle #1: Vitamins

We cannot forget the importance of daily vitamins. They help cover essential nutrients we don't get in our regular diets. As alluded to previously, the American diet is notorious for not having the complete nutrition the human body requires. Supplemental vitamins help fill that gap in our nutritional needs. Moreover, if a major crisis occurs, our diets will change. We may experience different deficiencies in our daily vitamin and mineral requirements. A good multivitamin will help to fill vital deficiencies that may appear in our nutrition.

It's fine to purchase the less-expensive, generic equivalent if it is available. I don't hesitate. It is what I always buy, and I am confident that the generic brands are quality tested and are extremely close to what the higher-priced, brand-name products offer. But if you are determined to purchase the brand name, go ahead. It's your money.

Take a look at the ingredient list on the different multivitamin products. Select one that has a good overall coverage of most of the vitamins and minerals. Remember, we need to get a two-year supply. Check the expiration dates on the bottles on the shelf, and get the best dates available. The better dates should be stocked toward the back.

Now that you have a good start on your daily vitamin and mineral needs, consider any additional supplement pills you may take. I highly recommend in addition to a good multivitamin also getting vitamin C, one thousand milligrams. I know that your multivitamin has vitamin C in it, but extra will not hurt you. Vitamin C is a great supplement for supporting your immune system. There is also evidence that it helps support your cardiovascular system and eye health and prevents skin wrinkling. A little too much vitamin C will not hurt you since any excess that your body cannot use is passed out through your kidneys. Do not go overboard and take the whole bottle. Too much of anything can harm you. *Moderation* is the key word here.

Now we need to turn to any other vitamin or mineral supplements you may take. If your doctor has suggested adding any other vitamins to your daily regimen, let's get them now.

Let's turn the cart around the corner and head into the next aisle.

Aisle #2: Pain Relievers

Here we have a wide assortment of choices. These are what I recommend, but if you have a personal preference for something else, go ahead and get it.

First, even though I like aspirin and think it truly is a miracle drug (it can be used for so many beneficial needs), it goes bad too quickly to be of much use. Ever opened up a bottle of aspirin and it smells just like vinegar? That is the chemical of aspirin, acetylsalicylic acid, breaking down into acetic acid. Technically, acetic acid is not bad for you; it is just vinegar. But if I'm going to take aspirin, I want aspirin. Despite the printed expiration date on aspirin, in my experience aspirin starts degrading right away and seems to last for only a few months. Also, aspirin is not recommended for use in children.

Acetaminophen and ibuprofen are good alternatives. Both relieve mild to moderate pain, and both can be used to bring down fevers. They are many hospitals' first drugs of choice for pain since they are so versatile. Both products can be used safely in children as long as you follow the manufacturer directions for dosage. Acetaminophen does not cause stomach problems, but taking too much ibuprofen *can* lead to ulcers. Ibuprofen has exceptional anti-inflammatory properties while acetaminophen does not. The maximum dosage of acetaminophen is four thousand milligrams per day, according to the FDA, and the maximum dosage of ibuprofen is thirty-two hundred milligrams per day. Too much acetaminophen can harm the liver while too much ibuprofen can harm the liver and kidneys.

Aisle #3: First Aid

You can never have too many first-aid products. Bandages, sterile pads, tape, and wraps do not go out of date. And no matter how much you have, you'll find that you always need more. There are so many different sizes of each of these products, you cannot possibly have them all unless you have a huge budget and plenty of storage space. You might also want to consider purchasing items such as vinyl gloves, masks, goggles for eye protection, surgical scissors, and non-mercury-based thermometers.

I recommend having at least two first aid kits around your home. In just one plastic case, you have all of the essentials for administering basic emergency first aid. They are very portable, and instead of having to try to remember to grab everything you need from your shelves, you can just grab the box and run. Make sure your emergency kits are in date because first-aid kits do have items inside that expire. Having a few boxes of individually packaged alcohol swabs in the kits is also a great idea. Your kits will be crucial after a major collapse, when medical personnel are in short supply.

Definitely have at least a few tubes (I have about ten) of antibiotic cream or ointment in your house. I cannot overemphasize the importance of treating any type of scratch or cut immediately. You don't want a major blood infection (sepsis) from a simple cut to ruin your survival potential. Topical antibiotics can nip a potentially life-threatening infection in the bud.

You will also need to have hydrocortisone 1 percent cream or ointment. Don't fool with the 0.5 percent strength. We want the strongest thing available over the counter. This is the best thing to treat topical skin rashes or insect bites. Do not substitute diphenhydramine (brand name: Benadryl®) cream for hydrocortisone. Diphenhydramine cream is not very effective. Finally, I recommend getting an antifungal cream or powder. The last thing you want when you are running through the woods or trudging along in wet weather is to get a nasty fungus infection on your toes.

Next, I would pick up a few bottles each of isopropyl (rubbing) alcohol, hydrogen peroxide, and povidone iodine (Betadine®). All three items are excellent at cleaning intact skin. Povidone iodine is a wonderful antiseptic and will disinfect wounds. Most surgical hospitals use it in their operating rooms. Isopropyl alcohol is another great antiseptic, but it will sting on open wounds and is extremely flammable. Hydrogen peroxide disinfects a wound by oxidizing (hence all the bubbles) and will not sting. Recent studies on all three products have shown that not only do they kill bacteria and other harmful organisms in an open wound, but they all have some harmful effects on the surrounding healthy tissue and may delay healing. Despite this observation, your primary objective is to kill the bacteria and prevent life-threatening infection.

Some additional products to consider are topical lice treatments and vaginal yeast-infection products. You might not need these medications now, but if you get them now you'll be grateful in the future when you do need them.

Aisle #4: Sun Products

Here we find our suntan products. Items like lip balm, sunscreen, and sunburn treatment (aloe, topical pain-relief products) line the shelves. You don't seem to think we need any of these products. You don't plan on any trips to the beach soon. Trust me—you will regret not getting some of these items now.

If a collapse of society occurs, then we will be spending more time outside than ever before. We'll be tending gardens, chopping wood, and feeding our livestock. All of these activities mean more exposure to sunlight. It doesn't matter where you live; as long as the sun is shining, you can get sunburned. Even people living in Alaska get sunburned.

Sunburn damages the upper layer of the skin. Not only is this painful, but it also compromises the integrity of the skin and may lead to infection. It is always better to prevent the burn before it occurs than it is to treat the bad outcomes later.

Aisle #5: Allergy

The most-important product in this section is diphenhydramine. Do not get the liquid or capsules but search for the more shelf stable tablets. Diphenhydramine can prevent serious medical emergencies arising from allergies. When your body has an allergy, your cells release histamine, the chemical that causes inflammation, redness, swelling, and itching. Diphenhydramine blocks this chemical. This medication can be used to help abort life-threatening allergic reactions to food, insect stings, and other environmental issues. It can also be used to help with seasonal allergies. Be aware that diphenhydramine, as its major side effect, causes drowsiness. This may be a bad side effect or a good one, depending on your circumstances. Most over-the-counter sleep aids contain diphenhydramine as their main active ingredient.

Aisle #6: Digestion/Nausea

A normal bowel movement is important to maintaining good health. Constipation can lead to blockages and malabsorption. On the other hand, diarrhea can quickly cause dehydration and electrolyte imbalances. Don't suffer from constipation now? You may in the future. If the end of society occurs, our diets will inevitably change. We may be hunting for our daily meals, and one side effect of a high-protein diet is constipation. Any change in diet can cause diarrhea. Additionally, eating spoiled food can cause severe diarrhea. Even moderate sickness can lead to either constipation or diarrhea.

For constipation, pick up some docusate sodium. This is the best natural medication to treat this problem. Remember to drink plenty of fluids to help wash the intestines out. Other products to consider are fiber bulking powders such as psyllium.

For bouts of diarrhea, pick up loperamide two milligrams. This is the best and strongest product available over the counter for diarrhea. In fact until recently, loperamide used to be by prescription only. For minor occurrences of diarrhea or loose stools, you may want just to let it happen. Diarrhea can be a way for the body to get rid of bad food in your stomach and intestines naturally. If not severe, and if it lasts for only a day, I would let it go untreated. However, if it is violent or lasts longer than one day, I would treat with loperamide. Either way you need to drink plenty of fluids, preferably something with replacement electrolytes.

Aisle #7: Cough, Cold, and Flu

There is a vast amount of products lining the shelves for cough, cold, and flu. There are too many variations between the products to offer advice on one product over another. Additionally, most of these products come in liquid form and are not shelf stable for long periods. I cannot recommend getting any products from this area right now. You might want to pick up a few multisymptom gelcaps and maybe a bottle or two of plain cough syrup. The problem with most of these products is that they use the "shotgun" approach to treating the symptoms of a cold. By "shotgun" I mean that the manufacturer packs the product full of ingredients to treat a wide spectrum of signs and symptoms, some of which you may not need. Then, with more ingredients come more side effects and other medication-related problems. We may have to go old school on colds and the flu by just toughing them out. That was the way we did it as children, before all of this medication was available on the market.

With this shopping list, you can easily acquire the basics for your medicine cabinet. You can add additional items as you go. Just remember to rotate and refresh your stock periodically.

Conclusion

THE ULTIMATE GOAL OF THIS book is to help you acquire and save as much prescription medication necessary to

I. maintain your medication supply until general order can be restored and manufacturer supply lines start producing your prescription medication again;

II. maintain your medication supply until you can successfully wean yourself off of the medication through lifestyle (eating and exercise) changes; or

III. maintain your medication supply until you can successfully find an alternative regimen to treat your medical condition.

I hope this book has been a good beginning to assist you in developing an action plan to maintain your health after an end-of-the-world event. Few people realize the importance of stockpiling their prescription medication. Lulled into a sense of complacency by the many myths that abound, they don't seem to realize the game of chance they are playing with their own well-being. Simple organization and planning can assure you of having at least a minimal level of prescription and nonprescription drugs at your disposal. Often overlooked but vitally important, having these products on hand may make the difference between perishing and surviving in a post-apocalyptic world.

www.ingramcontent.com/pod-product-compliance
Lightning Source LLC
Chambersburg PA
CBHW070839180526
45168CB00002B/882